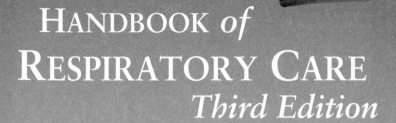

HANDBOOK *of*
RESPIRATORY CARE
Third Edition

D0807997

Robert L. Chatburn, MHHS, RRT-NPS, FAARC
Clinical Research Manager
Respiratory Institute
Cleveland Clinic
Adjunct Associate Professor
Department of Medicine
Lerner College of Medicine of Case Western Reserve University
Cleveland, Ohio

Eduardo Mireles-Cabodevila, MD
Director
Medial Intensive Care Unit
Assistant Professor
Division of Pulmonary and Critical Care Medicine
University of Arkansas for Medical Sciences
Little Rock, Arkansas

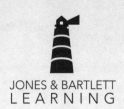

JONES & BARTLETT
LEARNING

World Headquarters
Jones & Bartlett Learning
40 Tall Pine Drive
Sudbury, MA 01776
978-443-5000
info@jblearning.com
www.jblearning.com

Jones & Bartlett Learning
Canada
6339 Ormindale Way
Mississauga, Ontario L5V 1J2
Canada

Jones & Bartlett Learning
International
Barb House, Barb Mews
London W6 7PA
United Kingdom

Jones & Bartlett Learning books and products are available through most bookstores and online booksellers. To contact Jones & Bartlett Learning directly, call 800-832-0034, fax 978-443-8000, or visit our website, www.jblearning.com.

Substantial discounts on bulk quantities of Jones & Bartlett Learning publications are available to corporations, professional associations, and other qualified organizations. For details and specific discount information, contact the special sales department at Jones & Bartlett Learning via the above contact information or send an email to specialsales@jblearning.com.

Copyright © 2011 by Jones & Bartlett Learning, LLC

All rights reserved. No part of the material protected by this copyright may be reproduced or utilized in any form, electronic or mechanical, including photocopying, recording, or by any information storage and retrieval system, without written permission from the copyright owner.

The authors, editor, and publisher have made every effort to provide accurate information. However, they are not responsible for errors, omissions, or for any outcomes related to the use of the contents of this book and take no responsibility for the use of the products and procedures described. Treatments and side effects described in this book may not be applicable to all people; likewise, some people may require a dose or experience a side effect that is not described herein. Drugs and medical devices are discussed that may have limited availability controlled by the Food and Drug Administration (FDA) for use only in a research study or clinical trial. Research, clinical practice, and government regulations often change the accepted standard in this field. When consideration is being given to use of any drug in the clinical setting, the health care provider or reader is responsible for determining FDA status of the drug, reading the package insert, and reviewing prescribing information for the most up-to-date recommendations on dose, precautions, and contraindications, and determining the appropriate usage for the product. This is especially important in the case of drugs that are new or seldom used.

Production Credits
Publisher: David Cella
Associate Editor: Maro Gartside
Production Director: Amy Rose
Senior Production Editor: Renée Sekerak
Marketing Manager: Grace Richards
Manufacturing and Inventory Control Supervisor: Amy Bacus
Composition: Northeast Compositors
Cover Design: Scott Moden
Cover Image: © Bocos Benedict/ShutterStock, Inc.
Printing and Binding: Malloy Incorporated
Cover Printing: Malloy Incorporated

Library of Congress Cataloging-in-Publication Data
Chatburn, Robert L.
  Handbook of respiratory care / Robert L. Chatburn, Eduardo Mireles-Cabodevila. -- 3rd ed.
    p. ; cm.
  Includes bibliographical references and index.
  ISBN 978-0-7637-8409-6 (pbk. : alk. paper)
  1. Respiratory therapy--Handbooks, manuals, etc. I. Mireles-Cabodevila, Eduardo. II. Title.
  [DNLM: 1. Respiratory Therapy--Handbooks. WF 39 C492h 2011]
  RC735.I5L68 2011
  616.2'0046--dc22
                                  2010023519

6048
Printed in the United States of America
14 13 12 11 10   10 9 8 7 6 5 4 3 2 1

Dedication

I would like to dedicate this book to three people. First is my daughter Maya, who has taught me how strength of spirit can carry you through any adversity. Second is my daughter Kendra, who has taught me that our world needs better planners who are inspired by a vision for social justice. Third is my mentor at the Cleveland Clinic, Dr. James K. Stoller, who taught me that faith in people is better than the "carrot or the stick."

RLC

To Marina, my wife, who endures, loves, guides, and nurtures. To my parents, Mario and Cristi, who taught me that it is not what they give you, it is what you do with it. To my sisters, for their persistence and joy. To my mentors, who had faith in me, and hopefully will never need to use the stick.

EMC

CONTENTS

APPENDIX **Reference Data 209**

Index 253

PREFACE

It has been 23 years since the *First Edition* of the *Handbook of Respiratory Care,* and 10 years since our last edition. During this period much has changed in the field of respiratory care, including advances in ventilation equipment, the development of evidence-based medicine, the universal presence of computers and the Internet in health care, and the standardization of nomenclatures and definitions. Yet much has not changed. Research and clinical practice still requires a reference standard, a source to obtain basic data that serves as foundation to research and clinical practice.

The *Handbook of Respiratory Care* is intended for both practicing clinicians and students wishing to have a summary of data not found in other textbooks. It is also intended for the clinician or researcher while reading an article, formulating research, or providing patient care. This edition has been adapted to be a companion of the contemporary clinician in the Internet era. Indeed, we now can obtain much information from the Internet; however, the *Handbook* represents years of collection of specific data that is not universally available. Nonetheless, it must be understood that this compilation, although intended to be global, is subject to change according to geographical location and practice variation.

The new edition was extensively revised to reflect current clinical needs in practice and research. We have devoted the first chapter to the most commonly used scores and definitions in respiratory and critical care research. Our goal is for the reader to have the ability to easily find what each score or definition entails and how it is calculated. It should also help as a starting point, as a source tool when attempting to design research. The pulmonary function chapter, Chapter 2, has been revised by Kevin McCarthy to reflect the recent changes in prediction equations in pulmonary function and exercise physiology. The chapters on physiology, gas therapy, and mathematical procedures were revised and updated. We added new concepts in physiology and acid–base physiology. All the chapters have new and easier to use tables, figures, and nomograms. The mechanical ventilation chapter now includes a simple-to-use method to classify and understand all the modes of mechanical ventilation. Finally, the appendix has grown in size and scope and now includes a collection of difficult-to-find concepts, figures, and classifications.

The *Handbook of Respiratory Care* compiles a wide variety of data from many sources in the fields of medicine, physics, mathematics, and engineering. It has been said that the key to knowledge is not in how many facts one may have memorized, but in knowing where to find them when needed. It is in this spirit that the *Third Edition* of the *Handbook of Respiratory Care* has been written. It is our hope that this edition becomes a good companion to the respiratory care clinicians and students attempting to navigate the overwhelming sea of information available.

RLC

EMC

■ CONTRIBUTING AUTHOR

Kevin McCarthy, RPFT
Technical Director/Manager
Pulmonary Function Laboratories
Cleveland Clinic, Respiratory Institute
Cleveland, Ohio

1

Scores and Definitions Used in Respiratory and Critical Care Research

Current articles use several scores and definitions to describe the population being studied. We present the scores as well as the original source. We also include the latest consensus in some definitions used in respiratory and critical care.

■ CHARLSON COMORBIDITY INDEX

Method for classifying comorbid conditions that might alter the risk of mortality for use in longitudinal studies. The one-year mortality rates for the different scores were 0: 12%; 1–2: 26%; 3–4: 52%; and greater than or equal to 5: 85%. The predicted risk of death from comorbid disease at a 10-year follow-up is 0: 8%; 1: 25%; 2: 48%; and greater than or equal to 3: 59%. Assigned weight for each patient's condition. The total equals the score.

- 1 point: Myocardial infarct, Congestive heart failure, Peripheral vascular disease, Cerebrovascular disease, Dementia, Chronic pulmonary disease, Connective tissue disease, Ulcer disease, Mild liver disease, and Diabetes
- 2 points: Hemiplegia, Moderate or severe renal disease, Diabetes with end-organ damage, Any tumor, Leukemia, and Lymphoma
- 3 points: Moderate or severe liver disease
- 6 points: Metastatic solid tumor, and AIDS

Data from Charlson, M. E. et al. *J Chronic Dis* 40 (1987), 373–383.

■ MCCABE CLASSIFICATION

Classification generated to obtain comparisons regarding the importance of host factors based on the severity of the underlying disease. *In parentheses we give the disease examples from the original article (McCabe, W. R. and Jackson, G. G. Arch of Int Med 110 (1962), 847–891). Evidently the prognosis for some has changed.*

- Category 1: Nonfatal disease (diabetes, genitourinary, gastrointestinal or obstetrical conditions)
- Category 2: Ultimately fatal disease (diseases estimated to become fatal within 4 years, e.g., aplastic anemia, metastatic carcinomas, cirrhosis, chronic renal disease)

Category 3: Rapidly fatal disease (acute leukemia, blastic relapse of chronic leukemia)

■ THE KNAUS CHRONIC HEALTH STATUS SCORE

Score used in the original APACHE article, and now used to describe baseline health status of the patients enrolled in studies.

Class A: Normal health status

Class B: Moderate activity limitation

Class C: Severe activity limitation due to chronic disease

Class D: Bedridden patient

Data from Knaus et al. *Crit Care Med* 9(8) (1981), 591–597.

■ GLASGOW COMA SCALE

(See Table 1–1.) Scale used to describe the neurological status of a patient, the neurological prognosis, and levels of brain injury. Points are added for each section.

Table 1-1 Glasgow Coma Scale

		Points
Eye opening	Spontaneous	4
	To voice	3
	To pain	2
	None	1
Verbal response	Oriented	5
	Confused	4
	Inappropriate words	3
	Incomprehensible words	2
	None	1
Motor response	Obeys commands	6
	Localizes	5
	Withdraws	4
	Flexion (decorticate)	3
	Extension (decerebrate)	2
	None	1

Data from Teasdale, G. M. and Jennet, B. *Lancet* 304 (1974), 81-84.

■ TRAUMA SCORE

(See Table 1–2.) A field scoring system in which values are correlated with probability of survival. Points are added from each category. A score of 1–5 points has a probability of survival of 0%; 6–7 points, 10%; 8–9 points, 22 to 37%; 10 points, 55%; 11 points, 71%; 12 points, 83%; and above 13 points, 90%.

Table 1-2 Trauma Score

Points	4	3	2	1	0
Respiratory Rate	10-24	25-35	>35	<10	Apnea
Respiratory Effort				Normal	Shallow or retractions
Systolic Blood Pressure	>90	70-90	50-69	<50	Not palpable
Capillary Refill			Normal	Delayed	None
Glasgow Coma Scale	14-15	11-13	8-10	5-7	3-4

Data from Champion, H. R. et al. *Crit Care Med* 9 (1981), 672-676.

■ REVISED TRAUMA SCORE (RTS)

(See Table 1–3.) A revised form of the trauma score used by the Trauma-Injury Scoring System (TRISS). It only uses three categories, for which a value is assigned. Each category value is multiplied by an assigned category weight, and the resultant values for each category are then added to obtain the RTS.

Table 1-3 Revised Trauma Score (RTS)

Points	4	3	2	1	0	Value	Weight[*]	Final Value
Respiratory Rate	10-29	>29	6-9	1-5	0		0.2908	
Systolic Blood Pressure	>89	76-89	50-75	1-49	0		0.7326	
Glasgow Coma Scale	13-15	9-12	6-8	4-5	3		0.9368	

[*]Multiply Value by Weight to get Final Value. Add all final values to obtain RTS scores.
Adapted from Champion, H. R. et al. *J Trauma* 29(5) (1989), 623-629.

■ PEDIATRIC TRAUMA SCORE

(See Table 1–4.) A score used to predict injury severity in pediatric patients. The sum of the points correlates with survival. Scores greater than 8 had a 0% mortality; between 0 and 8 had an increasing mortality. Scores below 0 had 100% mortality.

Table 1–4 Pediatric Trauma Score

Points	+2	+1	-1
Size	>20 kg	10-20 kg	<10 kg
Airway	Normal	Maintainable	Unmaintainable
Systolic Blood Pressure or Pulse	>90 mmHg	50-90 mmHg	<50 mmHg
	Pulse palpable wrist	Pulse palpable groin	No pulse palpable
Mental Status	Awake	Obtunded	Coma/ Decerebrate
Skeletal	None	Closed fracture	Open/Multiple fractures
Cutaneous	None	Minor	Major/ Penetrating

Adapted from Tepas, J. J. et al. *J. Trauma* 38 (1988), 425-429.

■ INJURY SEVERITY SCORE (ISS)

An anatomical scoring system that provides an overall score for patients with multiple injuries (Baker, et al. *J Trauma* 14 (1974), 187–196). Each injury is assigned an Abbreviated Injury Scale (AIS) score, allocated to one of six body regions (head, face, chest, abdomen, extremities, and external). Only the highest AIS score in each body region is used. The three most severely injured body regions have their score squared and added together to produce the ISS score.

The AIS ranges from 0 to 6, 0 being no injury, and 6 unsurvivable injury. The ISS values range from 0 to 75. A patient with an ISS score of 6 in any category automatically obtains the maximum ISS score (75). The AIS scores used are revised and published by the Association for the Advancement of Automotive Medicine.

■ TRAUMA-INJURY SEVERITY SCORE (TRISS)

A score that uses values from the ISS, the RTS, the patient age, and the type of injury to quantify the probability of survival (Boyd, C. R. et al. *J Trauma* 27(4) (1987), 370–378).

Age points: $\geq$55 years old = 1 point, otherwise 0 points.

TRISS (blunt): $b = -0.4499 + RTS \times 0.8085 +$ ISS $\times -0.0835 + $ (age points) $\times -1.7430$

or

TRISS (penetrating): $b = -2.5355 + RTS \times 0.9934 +$ ISS $\times -0.0651 +$ (age points) $\times -1.1360$

then

Probability of survival $= 1/(1 + e^b)$
Probability of death = 1 – probability of survival.

■ ACUTE PHYSIOLOGY AND CHRONIC HEALTH EVALUATION (APACHE II)

(See Tables 1–5 and 1–6.) Used as a clinical scoring system to classify the severity of illness. APACHE II uses the worst last values in the last 24 hours. To calculate the predicted death rate:

APACHE II SCORE = Acute Physiology Score + Age points + Chronic Health points

Ln $(R/1 - R) = -3.517 + ($ Apache II$) * 0.146 +$ Diagnostic Category Weight $+ 0.603$ if postemergency surgery.

Predicted Death Rate $= e^{Ln (R/1 - R)}/(1 + e^{Ln (R/1 - R)})$ where "e" is the base of natural logarithm, 2.718.

■ SEQUENTIAL ORGAN FAILURE ASSESSMENT (SOFA) SCORE

(See Table 1–7.) Score designed to describe the degree of organ dysfunction in critically ill patients.

Table 1-5 Acute Physiology and Chronic Health Evaluation (APACHE II)

APACHE II is used as a clinical scoring system to classify the severity of illness. It uses the worst last values in the last 24 hrs.

Physiologic Variable	Points								
	4	3	2	1	0	1	2	3	4
Temperature-rectal (°C)	≥41	39.9-40.9		38.5-38.9	36-38.4	34-35.9	32-33.9	30-31.9	≤29.9
Mean Arterial Pressure-mmHg	≥160	130-159	110-129		70-109		50-69		≤49
Heart Rate (ventricular response)	≥180	140-179	110-139		70-109		55-69	40-54	≤39
Respiratory Rate (total)	≥50	35-49		25-34	12-24	10-11	6-9		≤5
Oxygenation:									
a. FIO$_2$ ≥0.5 record A-aDO$_2$	≥500	350-499	200-349		<200				
b. FIO$_2$ <0.5 record only PaO$_2$					>70	61-70		55-60	<55
Arterial pH	≥7.7	7.6-7.69		7.5-7.59	7.33-7.49		7.25-7.32	7.15-7.24	<7.15
Serum HCO$_3$ use *only* if no ABG	≥52	41-51.9		32-40.9	22-31.9		18-21.9	15-17.9	<15
Serum Sodium (mMol/L)	≥180	160-179	155-159	150-154	130-149		120-129	111-119	≤110
Serum Potassium (mMol/L)	≥7	6-6.9		5.5-5.9	3.5-5.4	3-3.4	2.5-2.9		<2.5
Serum Creatinine (mg/100 mL) double point score if acute renal failure	≥3.5	2-3.4	1.5-1.9		0.6-1.4		<0.6		

(continued)

Table 1-5 Acute Physiology and Chronic Health Evaluation (APACHE II) (continued)

Physiologic Variable	Points							
	4	3	2	1	0	1	2	3	4
Hematocrit (%)	≥60		50-59.9	46-49.9	30-45.9		20-29.9		<20
White Blood Cells Count total/ mm³	≥40		20-39.9	15-19.9	3-14.9		1-2.9		<1
Glasgow Coma Score	Score = 15 minus actual Glasgow coma scale								

Total Acute Physiology Score: Add points from the 12 parameters above

Age	Points	Chronic Health Points: If patient has history of severe organ insufficiency or is
≤44	0	*Immunocompromised* assign points as follows:
45-54	2	**5 points** if nonoperative or emergency postoperative patients
55-64	3	**2 points** if elective postoperative patients
65-74	5	
≥75	6	

Definitions: Organ insufficiency or immunocompromised state must have been *evident prior* to hospital admission. **Liver failure:** Cirrhosis and portal hypertension or manifestations of liver failure. **Cardiovascular:** New York Heart Association Class IV. **Respiratory:** Chronic restrictive, obstructive, or vascular pulmonary disease with severe exercise restriction or documented chronic hypoxia hypercapnia, secondary polycytemia, severe pulmonary hypertension, or ventilator dependency. **Renal:** Chronic dialysis. **Immunocompromised:** Patient receiving therapy or has disease that suppresses resistance to infection. R = risk of hospital death.

Table 1-6 Diagnostic Categories Weight Leading to ICU Admission (APACHE II)

Nonoperative			
Respiratory Failure		**Trauma**	
Asthma/allergy	−2.108	Multiple trauma	−1.228
COPD	−0.367	Head injury	−0.517
Pulmonary edema (noncardiogenic)	−0.251	**Neurologic**	
Postrespiratory arrest	−0.168	Seizure disorder	−0.584
Aspiration/poisoning/toxic	−0.142	ICH/SDH/SAH	0.723
Pulmonary embolus	−0.128	**Other**	
Infection	0	Drug overdose	−3.353
Neoplasm	0.891	Diabetic ketoacidosis	−1.507
Cardiovascular Failure		GI Bleeding	0.334
Hypertension	−1.798	**If Not in One of These Groups, What System Was the Principal Reason for Admission?**	
Rythm disturbance	−1.368		
Congestive heart failure	−0.424		
Hemorrhagic shock/hypovolemia	0.493		
Coronary artery disease	−0.191	Metabolic/renal	−0.885
Sepsis	0.113	Respiratory	−0.890
Post cardiac arrest	0.393	Neurologic	−0.759
Cardiogenic shock	−0.259	Cardiovascular	0.470
Dissecting thoracic/abdominal aneurysm	0.731	Gastrointestinal	0.501
Postoperative			
		If Postemergency Surgery	
Multiple trauma	−1.684	−1.081	
Admission due to chronic cardio-vascular disease	−1.376	−0.773	
Peripheral vascular surgery	−1.315	−0.712	
Heart valve surgery	−1.261	−0.658	
Craniotomy for neoplasm	−1.245	−0.642	
Renal surgery for neoplasm	−1.204	−0.601	
Renal transplant	−1.042	−0.439	
Head trauma	−0.955	−0.352	
Thoracic surgery for neoplasm	−0.802	−0.199	
Craniotomy for ICH/SDH/SAH	−0.788	−0.185	
Laminectomy and other spinal cord surgery	−0.699	−0.096	
Hemorrhagic shock	−0.682	−0.079	

(continued)

Table 1-6 Diagnostic Categories Weight Leading to ICU Admission (APACHE II cont.)

	Postoperative	
		If Postemergency Surgery
GI bleeding	−0.617	−0.014
GI surgery for neoplasm	−0.248	0.355
Respiratory insufficiency	−0.140	0.463
GI perforation/obstruction	0.060	0.663
If Not in One of the Above, What System Led to ICU Admission Postsurgery?		
Neurologic	−1.150	−0.574
Cardiovascular	−0.797	−0.194
Respiratory	−0.610	−0.007
Gastrointestinal	−0.613	−0.01
Metabolic/renal	−0.196	0.407

Adapted from Knaus, W. A. et al. *Crit Care Med* 13 (1985), 818-829.

Table 1-7 Sequential Organ Failure Assessment (SOFA) Score

Points	1	2	3	4
Respiration Pao_2/Fio_2, mmHg	<400	<300	<200	<100
Coagulation Platelets × 10^3/mm³	<150	<100	<50	<20
Liver Bilirubin, mg/dl	1.2-1.9	2.0-5.9	6.0-11.9	>12
Cardiovascular *Hypotension*[*]	MAP <70	Dopamine ≤5 or dobutamine (any dose)	Dopamine >5 or epinephrine ≤0.1 or norepinephrine ≤0.1	Dopamine >15 or epinephrine >0.1 or norepinephrine >0.1
Central Nervous System Glasgow Coma Score	13-14	10-12	6-9	<6
Renal Creatinine mg/dl or Urine Output	1.2-1.9	2.0-3.4	3.5-4.9 or <500 mL/day	>5 or <200 mL/day

[*]Vasopressors agents administered for at least 1 hr (μg/kg·min)
Adapted from Vincent, J. L. et al. *Int Care Med* 22 (1996), 707-710.

■ MULTIPLE ORGAN DYSFUNCTION (MOD) SCORE

(See Table 1–8.) Score designed to describe the degree of organ dysfunction in critically ill patients. It correlates with intensive care and hospital mortality and intensive care unit length of stay as originally described.

Table 1–8 Multiple Organ Dysfunction Score

Organ System	0	1	2	3	4
Respiratory Pao_2/Fio_2	>300	226-300	151-225	76-150	≤75
Renal Serum creatinine μmol/L (mg/dl)	≤100 (1.1)	101-200 (1.1-2.3)	201-350 (2.3-4)	351-500 (4-5.7)	>500 (5.7)
Liver Serum bilirubin μmol/L (mg/dl)	≤20 (1.2)	21-60 (1.2-3.5)	61-120 (3.6-7)	121-240 (7.1-14)	>240 (14)
Cardiovascular Pressure-adjusted heart rate*	≤10	10.1-15	15.1-20	20.1-30	>30
Hematologic Platelet count mL 10^{-3}	>120	81-120	51-80	21-50	≤20
Neurologic Glasgow coma score**	15	13-14	10-21	7-9	≤6

*Pressure-adjusted heart rate = (heart rate × right atrial pressure)/mean arterial pressure.
**For patients receiving sedation or muscle relaxants normal brain function is assumed unless there is evidence of altered mentation.

MOD Score	Intensive Care Unit Mortality	Hospital Mortality	Intensive Care Unit Stay (days)
0	0%	0%	2
1-4	1-2%	7%	3
5-8	3-5%	16%	6
9-12	25%	50%	10
13-16	50%	70%	17
17-20	75%	82%	21
21-24	100%	100%	n.a.

Adapted from Marshall, J. C. et al. *Crit Care Med* 23 (1995), 1638-1652.

■ SIMPLIFIED ACUTE PHYSIOLOGY SCORE (SAPS II) AND EXPANDED VERSION

(See Table 1–9.) Score to calculate to probability of hospital mortality. The score revised in 2005 is referred to as the expanded version. The score uses the worst value (the one that gives the most points) in last 24 hours.

Table 1-9 Simplified Acute Physiology Score (SAPS II) and Expanded Version

SAPS II	0 points	Abnormal value points			
Age, years	<40	40-59 7 points	60-69 12 points	70-74 15 points	75-79 16 points	≥ 80 18 points
Heart rate, beats/min	70-119	40-69 2 points	120-159 4 points	≥ 160 7 points	< 40 11 points	
Systolic Blood Pressure, mmHg	100-199	>200 2 points	70 -99 5 points	≤ 70 13 points		
Body Temperature, °C	<39	≥ 39 3 points				
Only if on Mechanical Ventilation* Pao$_2$ mmHg/ Fio$_2$		≥ 200 6 points	100-199 9 points	<100 11 points		
Urinary Output, L/day	≥ 1	0.5-0.9 4 points	< 05 11 points			
Blood Urea Nitrogen, mg/dL	<28	28-83 6 points	≥ 84 10 points			
White Blood Cell Count, mm^3	1-19.9	≥ 20 3 points	<1.0 12 points			
Potassium, mEq/L	3-4.9	< 3 or ≥ 5 3 points				
Sodium, mEq/L	125-144	≥145 1 point	< 125 5 points			
Bicarbonate, mEq/L	≥20	15-19 3 points	< 15 6 points			
Bilirubin, mg/dl	<4	4-5.9 4 points	≥ 6 9 points			
Glasgow Coma Score	14-15	11-13 5 points	9 - 10 7 points	6 - 8 13 points	<6 26 points	

(continued)

Table 1-9 Simplified Acute Physiology Score (SAPS II) and Expanded Version (cont.)

SAPS II	0 points	Abnormal value points	
Chronic Disease		Metastatic cancer 9 points Hematological malignancy 10 points AIDS 17 points	**SAPS II SCORE: add worst value for last 24 hours**
Type of Admission	Scheduled surgical	Medical 6 points Unscheduled surgical 8 points	

*Mechanical ventilation includes the use of continuous positive airway pressure (CPAP).

SAPS II expanded		
	Value	Points
Age, years	<40	0
	40-59	0.1639
	60-69	0.2739
	70-79	0.369
	>79	0.6645
Sex	Male	0.2083
	Female	0
Length of Hospital Stay Before ICU Admission	<24 hours	0
	1 day	0.0986
	2 days	0.1944
	3-9 days	0.5284
	>9 days	0.9323
Patient's Location Before ICU	Emergency room or mobile emergency unit	0
	Ward in same hospital	0.2606
	Other hospital	0.3381
Clinical Category	Medical patient	0.6555
	Other	0
Intoxication	No	1.6693
	Yes	0
SAPS II (Expanded) = 0.0742 × SAPS II score + the sum of the expanded variables		

To calculate the predicted mortality:

Logit = $-14.4761 + 0.0844 \times$ SAPS II(expanded) $+ 6.6158 \times$ log[SAPS II(expanded) + 1]

then

predicted mortality $= e^{(Logit)}/[1 + e^{(Logit)}]$

Adapted from Le Gall, J. R. et al. *JAMA* 270 (1993), 2957-2963; and Le Gall, J. R. et al. *Critical Care* (2005), R645-R652.

■ PEDIATRIC RISK OF MORTALITY (PRISM)

(See Table 1–10.) Score designed to calculate the mortality risk in the pediatric intensive care unit. Developed from the original Physiologic Stability

Table 1-10 Pediatric Risk of Mortality (PRISM)

	Infants (<1 year old)	Children	All ages	Score
Systolic Blood Pressure, mmHg	55-65 or 130-160	65-75 or 150-200		2
	40-54 or >160	50-64 or >200		6
	<40	<50		7
Diastolic Blood Pressure, mmHg			>110	6
Heart Rate, beats per minute	<90 or >160	<80 or >150		4
Respiratory Rate, breaths per minute	61-90	51-70		1
	apnea or >90	apnea or >70		5
Pao$_2$/Fio$_2$			200-300	2
			<200	3
Paco$_2$ torr			51-65	1
			>65	5
Glasgow Coma Score			<8	6
Pupillary Reaction			unequal or dilated	4
			fixed and dilated	10
PT/PTT			1.5 × control	2
Total Bilirubin, mg/dl			>3.5 (>1 month old)	6
Potassium, mEq/L			3-3.5 or 6.5-7.5	1
			<3.0 or >7.5	5
Calcium, mg/dL			7-8 or 12-15	2
			<7 or >15	6
Glucose, mg/dL			40-60 or 250-400	4
			<40 or >400	8
Bicarbonate, mEq/L			<16 or >32	3

Adapted from Pollack, M. M. et al. *Crit Care Med* 16 (1988), 1110-1116.

Index. Values are measured during the first 24 hours after intensive care admission.

First, calculate the risk of death (r).

$$r = (0.207 \times \text{PRISM}) - [0.005 \times (\text{age in months})] - 0.433 \times 1$$
$$(\text{if postoperative}) - 4.782$$

Then

$$\text{predicted death rate} = e^r/(1 + e^r)$$

■ PEDIATRIC INDEX OF MORTALITY II (PIM II)

(See Table 1–11.) Score used to estimate mortality risk from data obtained for each variable measured within the period from the time of first contact (anywhere by an ICU doctor) to 1 hour after arrival to the intensive care unit.

Table 1–11 Pediatric Index of Mortality II (PIM II)

Variable		Value
a	Systolic blood pressure, mmHg	MV if unknown = 120 cardiac arrest = 0 shock with unmeasurable SBP = 30
b	Pupillary reactions to bright light	>3 mm and both fixed = 1 other or unknown = 0
c	($F_{IO_2} \times 100$)/Pa_{O_2}, mmHg	MV if unknown = 0
d	Base excess in arterial or capillary blood, mmol/L	MV if unknown = 0
e	Mechanical ventilation at any time during the first hour in ICU	no = 0, yes = 1
f	Elective admission to ICU	no = 0, yes = 1
g	Recovery from surgery or a procedure is the main reason for ICU admission	no = 0, yes = 1
h	Admitted following cardiac bypass	no = 0, yes = 1

(continued)

Table 1-11 Pediatric Index of Mortality II (PIM II) (continued)

Variable		Value
i	**High-risk diagnosis is the main reason for ICU admission**	no = 0, yes = 1
	Cardiac arrest preceding ICU admission	
	Severe combined immune deficiency	
	Leukemia or lymphoma after first induction	
	Spontaneous cerebral hemorrhage	
	Cardiomyopathy or myocarditis	
	Hypoplastic left heart syndrome	
	HIV infection	
	Liver failure is the main reason for ICU admission	
	Neurodegenerative disorder	
j	**Low-risk diagnosis is the main reason for ICU admission**	no = 0, yes = 1
	Asthma	
	Bronchiolitis	
	Croup	
	Obstructive sleep apnea	
	Diabetic ketoacidosis	

MV = Measured value. Enter the value for each variable in the equation.
Adapted from Slater et al. *Int Care Med* 29 (2003), 278-285.

$$\text{PIM2} = \{0.01395 \times [\text{absolute } (a - 120)]\} + (3.0791 \times b) + (0.2888 \times c)$$
$$+ (0.104 \times \text{absolute } d) + (1.3352 \times e) - (0.9282 \times f) - (1.0244 \times g) +$$
$$(0.7507 \times h) + (1.6829 \times i) - (1.5770 \times j) - 4.8841$$

Then

$$\text{probability of death} = e^{\text{PIM2}}/(1 + e^{\text{PIM2}})$$

■ APGAR SCORE

(See Table 1–12.) Score that is assessed at 1 and 5 minutes after delivery. It may be repeated at 5-minute intervals for infants with 5-minute scores <7. Add points for each category.

Table 1-12 Apgar Score

Sign	0	1	2
Heart Rate	Absent	<100 bpm	>100 bpm
Respiratory Effort	Absent	Irregular, shallow	Good, crying
Muscle Tone	Limp	Some flexion of extremities	Active motion
Reflex Irritability	No response	Grimace	Cry
Color	Blue, pale	Body pink, extremities blue	Completely pink

Data from Apgar, V. *Anesth Analg* 32 (1953), 260.

Interpretation:

10: Best possible condition.

7–9: Adequate, no treatment.

4–6: Infant requires close observation and intervention such as suctioning.

<4: Infant requires immediate intervention such as intubation and further examination.

■ SILVERMAN SCORE

(See Figure 1–1.)

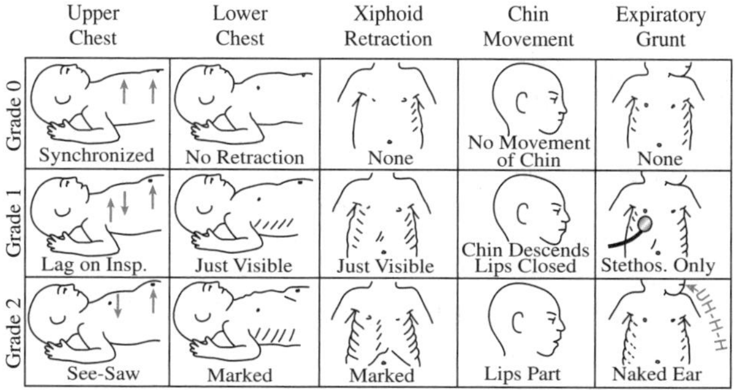

Figure 1-1 Silverman score. (Adapted from Silverman, W. A. and Andersen, D. H. *Pediatrics* 17 (1956), 1-10.).

Evaluates: Retractions, nasal flaring, and grunting.

Use: Evaluates respiratory distress in newborns.

Interpretation: Zero indicates no respiratory distress; 10 indicates severe respiratory distress; 7 or greater indicates impending respiratory failure.

■ NEWBORN RESPIRATORY DISTRESS SCORING (RDS) SYSTEM

(See Table 1–13.) The sum of all the individual scores. Clinical RDS = score ≥4 (overall mortality 25%); score ≥8 = severe respiratory distress with impending failure (65% mortality).

Table 1-13 Newborn Respiratory Distress Scoring (RDS) System[*]

RDS Score	0	1	2
Cyanosis	None	In-room air	In 40% FIO_2
Retractions	None	Mild	Severe
Grunting	None	Audible with stethoscope	Audible without stethoscope
Air Entry (crying)[*]	Clear	Delayed or decreased	Barely audible
Respiratory Rate (min)	60	60-80	>80 or apneic episodes

[*]Air entry represents the quality of the inspiratory breath sounds as heard in the midaxillary line.
Adapted from Downes, J. J. et al. *Clin Pediatr* (Phila) 9(6) (1970), 325-331.

■ SEPSIS DEFINITION

In an effort to standardize patients into categories of sepsis, a classification has been widely adopted. Although it has limitations, when revised 10 years later the same definitions stand with some new expansions. (From Bone, R. C. et al. *CHEST* 101 (1992), 1644–1655 and Levy, M. M. et al. *Critical Car Med* 31 (2003), 1250–1256.)

Systemic Inflammatory Response Syndrome

More than one of the following:

1. Body temperature greater than 38°C
2. Heart rate greater than 90 beats per minute

3. Tachypnea (respiratory rate >20 breaths per minute) or hyperventilation (P_{ACO_2} <32 mmHg at sea level)
4. White blood cell count ≥12000 or ≤4000/cu mm.

Infection

Pathologic process caused by the invasion of normally sterile tissue or fluid or body cavity by pathogenic or potentially pathogenic microorganism.

Sepsis

Clinical syndrome defined by the presence of both infection (suspected or confirmed) and systemic inflammatory response. *Diagnostic criteria for sepsis in the pediatric population* are signs and symptoms of inflammation plus infection with hyper- or hypothermia (rectal temperature >38.5 or <35°C), tachycardia and one of the following indications of organ dysfunction: altered mental status, hypoxemia, increased serum lactate level, or bounding pulses.

Severe Sepsis

Sepsis complicated by organ dysfunction. May use the SOFA score or the MOD score (see above) to define organ dysfunction.

Septic Shock

Acute circulatory failure characterized by persistent arterial hypotension unexplained by other causes. *Septic shock in pediatric patients* is defined as tachycardia with signs of decreased organ perfusion (decreased peripheral pulses compared with central pulses, altered mental status, capillary refill >2 s, mottled or cool extremities, or decreased urine output).

Hypotension

Systolic blood pressure below 90 mmHg (in children <2 SD below normal for their age), a mean arterial pressure <60 mmHg, or a reduction in systolic blood pressure of >40 mmHg from baseline despite adequate volume resuscitation.

■ 2001 EXPANDED DIAGNOSTIC CRITERIA FOR SEPSIS

Infection (defined as a pathologic process induced by a microorganism), documented or suspected, and some of the following:

General Variables

Fever (core temperature >38.3°C)

Hypothermia (core temperature <36°C)

Heart rate >90 min or >2 SD above the normal value for age

Tachypnea

Altered mental status

Significant edema or positive fluid balance (>20 mL/kg over 24 h)

Hyperglycemia (plasma glucose >120 mg/dL) in the absence of diabetes

Inflammatory Variables

Leukocytosis (white blood cell count >12,000 μL)

Leukopenia (white blood cell count <4000 μL)

Normal white blood cell count with >10% immature forms

Plasma C-reactive protein >2 SD above the normal value

Plasma procalcitonin >2 SD above the normal value

Hemodynamic Variables

Arterial hypotension (systolic blood pressure <90 mm Hg, mean arterial pressure <70, or a systolic blood pressure decrease >40 mm Hg in adults or <2 SD below normal for age)

Mixed venous oxygen saturation >70%

Cardiac index >3.5 Lmin · m^2

Organ Dysfunction Variables

Arterial hypoxemia (P_{AO_2}/F_{IO_2} <300)

Acute oliguria (urine output <0.5 mL/kg/h or 45 mmol/L for at least 2 h)

Creatinine increase >0.5 mg/dL

Coagulation abnormalities (INR >1.5 or aPTT >60 s)

Ileus (absent bowel sounds)

Thrombocytopenia (platelet count <100,000 μL)

Hyperbilirubinemia (plasma total bilirubin >4 mg/dL)

Tissue Perfusion Variables

Hyperlactatemia (>1 mmol/L)

Decreased capillary refill or mottling

■ VASOPRESSOR SCORE (INOTROPIC SCORE, CATHECHOLAMINE INDEX)

Score used to describe the dose of vasopressors used.

$$\text{inotropic score} = (\text{dopamine dose} \times 1) + (\text{dobutamine dose} \times 1) + (\text{adrenaline dose} \times 100) + (\text{noradrenaline dose} \times 100) + (\text{phenylephrine dose} \times 100)$$

$$\text{vasopressor dependency index} = \text{inotropic score}/\text{MAP}$$

Data from Cruz, D. N. et al. *JAMA* 301(23) (2009), 2445–2452.

■ ACUTE RESPIRATORY DISTRESS SYNDROME DEFINITION

As defined by Bernard, et al. (*Am J Respir Crit Care Med* 149 (1994), 818–824), all of the following criteria must be present

- ■ Acute onset
- ■ PaO_2/FIO_2 ≤200 mmHg (ARDS)
- ■ PaO_2/FIO_2 ≤300 mmHg (acute lung injury, ALI)
- ■ Bilateral infiltrates on chest radiograph consistent with pulmonary edema
- ■ Pulmonary artery occlusion pressure ≤18 mmHg or no clinical evidence of left atrial hypertension

■ LUNG INJURY SCORE (MURRAY SCORE)

(See Table 1–14.) Designed to characterize the presence and extent of a pulmonary damage, the lung injury score was part of a three-component definition in the original paper. The lung injury score was used as the definition for ARDS (Score >2.5), but it is still used rather to characterize the severity of lung disease in clinical trials.

Table 1-14 Lung Injury Score (Murray Score)

| | SCORE | | | | |
	0	1	2	3	4
Chest Radiograph Number of Quadrants with Alveolar Consolidation	None	1	2	3	4
Hypoxemia Pao_2/Fio_2	≥ 300	225-299	175-224	100-174	<100
PEEP cmH_2O	≤ 5	6-8	9-11	12-14	≥ 15
Lung Compliance $mL/cm\ H_2O$	≥ 80	60-79	40-59	20-39	≤ 19

Add individual scores for each category and then divide by the number of components used. (i.e., not all patients have all measurements).
Adapted from Murray, et al. *Am Rev Respir Dis* 138 (1988), 720-723.

■ VENTILATOR-FREE DAYS

The number of ventilator-free days is used to evaluate the effects of therapies in critical care. This number combines the effects of mortality and the duration of mechanical ventilation in patients who survive. It assumes that any therapy that decreases duration of mechanical ventilation in patients who survive also increases the number of patients that survive. The number is calculated as

> ventilator-free days = number of days from day 1 to day 28
> on which a patient breathed without assistance (if the period
> of unassisted breathing lasted at least 48 consecutive hours).

If patient dies or requires more than 28 days of mechanical ventilation, the value is 0. (From Schoenfeld, D. A. et al. *Crit Care Med* 30 (2002), 1772–1777.)

■ PNEUMONIA DEFINITIONS

The following definitions are from the American Thoracic Society and Infectious Diseases Society of America in 2005 (*Am J Respir Crit Care Med* 171 (2005), 388–416).

Community-Acquired Pneumonia

Pneumonia occurring within 48 hours of admission in patients with no criteria for healthcare-associated pneumonia.

Ventilator-Associated Pneumonia

- Pneumonia occurring >48 hours after endotracheal intubation.
- Defined as a new lung infiltrate on chest radiography plus at least two of the following: fever, 38°C, leukocytosis or leukopenia, and purulent secretions.

Hospital-Acquired Pneumonia

Pneumonia occurring ≥48 hours after hospital admission

Risk factors for multidrug resistant bacteria:

- Antibiotic therapy within 90 days of infection.
- Current hospitalization of ≥5 days.
- High frequency of antibiotic resistance in community or specific hospital unit.
- Immunosuppressive disease or therapy.
- Presence of healthcare-associated pneumonia risk factors for multidrug resistant bacteria.

Healthcare-Associated Pneumonia

Pneumonia occurring ≤48 hours of admission in patients with any risk factor for multidrug resistant bacteria as cause of infection:

- Hospitalization for ≥2 days in an acute-care facility within 90 days of infection.
- Nursing home or long-term acute-care facility resident.
- Antibiotic therapy, chemotherapy, or wound care in last 30 days.
- Hemodialysis at a hospital or clinic.
- Home infusion therapy or wound care.
- Family member with infection due to a multidrug resistant bacteria.

■ CLINICAL PULMONARY INFECTION SCORE

(See Table 1–15.) Originally described by Pugin et al. (*Am Rev Resp Dis* 143 (1991), 1121–1129) and later modified by Singh et al. (*AJRCCM* 162 (2000), 505–511). A score developed to establish a numerical value of clinical, radiographic, and laboratory markers for pneumonia. Scores above 6 suggest pneumonia (specificity and sensitivity have been consistently less than in initial validation study). Singh et al. showed that some patients with a low clinical suspicion of ventilator-associated pneumonia (CPIS ≤6) can have antibiotics safely discontinued after 3 days, if the subsequent course suggests that the probability of pneumonia is still low. (See also Table 1–16.)

Table 1-15 Clinical Pulmonary Infection Score

Score	0	1	2
Temperature	≥36.5 and ≤38.4	≥38.5 and ≤38.9	≥39 or ≤36.4
Blood Leukocytes 10^3 mm^3	≥4 and ≤11	<4 or >12	
Tracheal Secretions	None	Nonpurulent	Purulent
Oxygenation Pao$_2$/Fio$_2$, mmHg	>240 or ARDS*		≤240 and no ARDS
Chest Radiography	No opacity	Diffuse (patchy) opacities	Localized opacity
Progression of Radiographic Opacities	No progression		progression (after HF** and ARDS excluded)
Culture of Tracheal Aspirate	Pathogenic bacteria cultured in rare/few quantities or no growth	Pathogenic bacteria cultured in moderate or heavy quantity	

Add a point (+1) if: Bands are >50% or same pathogenic bacteria seen on Gram stain.

*ARDS (Acute Respiratory Distress Syndrome) defined as Pao$_2$/Fio$_2$ 200, PAOP <18 mmHg and acute bilateral infiltrates.

**HF: heart failure.

Adapted from Singh et al. *AJRCCM* 162 (2000), 505-511.

Table 1-16 Clinical Criteria for the Diagnosis of Pneumonia as Defined by the National Nosocomial Infection Surveillance System

Radiographic
Two or more serial chest radiographs with new or progressive and persistent infiltrate or cavitation or consolidation (one radiograph is sufficient in patients without underlying cardiopulmonary disease)
Clinical
One of the following:
Fever >38°C (100.4°F) with no other recognized cause
WBC count <4,000/μL or >12,000 μL
For adults >70 yr old, altered mental status with no other recognized cause
And at least two of the following:
New-onset purulent sputum or change in character of sputum, or increase in respiratory secretions or suctioning requirements
New-onset or worsening cough, dyspnea, or tachypnea
Rales or bronchial breath sounds
Worsening gas exchange, increased oxygen requirements, increased ventilatory support
Microbiology (optional)
Positive culture result (one): blood (unrelated to other source), pleural fluid, quantitative culture by BAL or PSB, >5% BAL-obtained cells contain intracellular bacteria

BAL: Bronchoalveolar lavage, PSB: Protected specimen brush
From CDC. *NNIS Criteria for Determining Nosocomial Pneumonia.* Atlanta, GA: U.S. Department of Health and Human Services, CDC, 2003. Prozencaski. *CHEST,* 2006; 130:597-604.

■ DEFINITIONS FOR WEANING AND LIBERATION OF MECHANICAL VENTILATION

Multiple terms and definitions are used indistinctly to describe the process of discontinuation of mechanical ventilation. The process of freeing a patient from ventilator assistance is often termed weaning (which for some includes the process of extubation). We favor the term liberation or discontinuation to describe the cessation of ventilator support. Table 1–18 shows the latest multisociety attempt to define weaning/liberation of mechanical ventilation.

Table 1-17 Definitions for Weaning and Liberation of Mechanical Ventilation

Weaning success: is the extubation and the absence of ventilatory support for the following 48 h

Weaning failure: is one of the following: (1) failed spontaneous breathing trial; or (2) reintubation and/or resumption of ventilator support following successful extubation; or (3) death within 48 h following extubation

Simple weaning: Patients who proceed from initiation of weaning to successful extubation on the first attempt

Difficult weaning: Patients who fail initial weaning and require up to three spontaneous breathing trials, or as long as 7 days from the first attempt to achieve successful weaning

Prolonged weaning: Patients who fail at least three weaning attempts or require more than 7 days of weaning after the first spontaneous breathing trial

Failed spontaneous breathing trial:

Subjective criteria: Agitation, anxiety, depressed mental status, diaphoresis, cyanosis, increased accessory muscle activity, facial signs of distress and dyspnea

Objective criteria: $PaO_2 \leq 50\text{-}60$ mmHg on $FIO_2 \geq 0.5$ or $SaO_2 < 90\%$; $PaCO_2 > 50$ mmHg or an increase in $PaCO_2 > 8$ mmHg; pH < 7.32 or a decrease in pH ≥ 0.07 pH units; shallow breathing index (respiratory rate/tidal volume) > 105 breaths/min/L; respiratory rate > 35 breaths/min or increased by $> 50\%$; heart rate > 140 beats/min or increased by $\geq 20\%$; systolic blood pressure > 180 mmHg or increased by $\geq 20\%$ or < 90 mmHg; or cardiac arrhythmias

Data from Boles, J. M. et al. *Eur Respir J* 29 (2007), 1033-1056.

■ INTUBATION DIFFICULTY SCALE

(See Table 1–18.) Quantitative score used to evaluate intubation difficulty, conditions, and techniques.

■ WELLS SCORE: PULMONARY EMBOLISM

The original interpretation of results of the Wells score for pulmonary embolism was modified for the Christopher study. Both are presented here.

Original Score

■ Symptoms of deep venous thrombosis (DVT): Leg swelling, pain with palpation (3 points).

■ No alternative diagnosis better explains the illness (3 points).

Table 1-18 Intubation Difficulty Scale

	Score			
	0	1	2	3
Number of Attempts	+1 for each attempt			
Number of Operators	+1 for each operator			
Number of Alternative Techniques	+1 for each change (blade, position, equipment, aproach, technique)			
Glotic Exposure*	Complete visualization of the vocal cords	Inferior portion of the glottis	Only the epiglottis	Nonvisualized epiglottis
Lifting Force Required	Little effort	Increased effort		
Laryngeal Pressure	Not applied**	Applied		
Vocal Cord Mobility	Abduction	Adduction		

*Use Cormack's visual grade (*Anesthesiology* 39 (1984), 1105-1111).

**"Sellick maneuver is used to prevent aspiration gastric contents and gives no points. Add all points to obtain total score. If unable to intubate, use total value previous to abandoning effort.

Adapted from Adnet, et al. *Anesthesiology* 87(6) (1997), 1290-1297.

- Tachycardia with pulse >100 (1.5 points).
- Immobilization (≥3 days) or surgery in the previous four weeks (1.5 points).
- Prior history of DVT or pulmonary embolism (1.5 points).
- Presence of hemoptysis (1 point).
- Presence of malignancy (1 point).

   Results: 7–12 points: High probability

   2–6 points: Moderate probability

   0–1 points: Low Probability

Modified Score

Use original criteria.

   Results: More than 4 points: Pulmonary embolism likely

   Less than 4 points: Pulmonary embolism unlikely

Data from Wells, P. S. et al. *Thrombosis and Haemostasis* 83 (2000), 416–420; and van Belle, A. et al. *JAMA* 295 (2006), 172.

■ WELLS SCORE: DEEP VENOUS THROMBOSIS (DVT)

The original Wells score and its interpretation were modified in a later article. Both are presented here.

Original Score

- Paralysis, paresis, or recent orthopedic casting of lower extremity (1 point).
- Recently bedridden (≥3 days) or major surgery within past 4 weeks (1 point).
- Localized tenderness in deep vein system (1 point).
- Swelling of entire leg (1 point).
- Calf swelling 3 cm greater than other leg (measured 10 cm below the tibial tuberosity) (1 point).
- Pitting edema greater in the symptomatic leg (1 point).
- Collateral nonvaricose superficial veins (1 point).

- Active cancer or cancer treated within 6 months (1 point).
- Alternative diagnosis more likely than DVT (−2 points).

   Results: 3–8 points: High probability of DVT

   1–2 points: Moderate probability

   −2–0 points : Low Probability

Modified Score

Add this criteria to the original.

- Previous documented DVT (1 point).

   Results: 2 or > points: DVT likely

   1 or less points: DVT unlikely

Data from Wells, P. S. et al. *Lancet* 350 (1997), 1795–1798; and Wells, P. S., Anderson, D. R., Rodger, M., et al. *N Engl J Med* 349 (2003), 179–1227.

CHAPTER

2

Pulmonary Function

Kevin McCarthy, RPFT

The following prediction equations are compiled from the works of many scientific investigators. Recent work has shown that Caucasians have significantly higher values for lung function than nearly every other ethnic group studied. Typical normal values for spirometry volumes in non-Caucasian individuals range from 85%–88% of the Caucasian predicted value. The NHANES III (Hankinson et al.) predicted set for spirometry provides specific regression equations for Caucasians, African-Americans, and Mexican-Americans; Caucasian values are presented here. Readers are directed to the reference to see these specific reference equations.

Tidal Volume (VT)

The volume of gas inspired or expired during one respiration cycle. Prediction equations are shown in Table 2–1.

Table 2-1 Tidal Volume (VT)

Infant	V_T = 7.1 mL/kg
Child	V_T = 7.5 mL/kg
Male adult	V_T = 7.8 mL/kg
Female adult	V_T = 6.6 mL/kg

Respiratory Rate or Frequency (f)

The number of respiratory cycles per unit of time, usually 1 minute. Prediction equations for respiratory frequency are shown in Table 2–2.

Table 2-2 Respiratory Rate or Frequency (f)

Age (6-25 yr)	f (bpm) = 30.9 − 0.80 age (years)
Age (25-80 yr)	f (bpm) = 7.07 + 0.16 age (years)

Alveolar Ventilation ($\dot{V}_A$)

The effective rate at which air enters the region of the lungs that participates in gas exchange. The calculation of alveolar ventilation is

$$\dot{V}_A = f \times (V_T - V_D)$$

where V_D = physiologic dead space volume.

Typical values for the preceding and more are shown in Table 2–3.

Table 2-3 Typical Values for Tidal Volume (V_T), Frequency (f), Minute Volume ($\dot{V}_E$), Dead Space (V_D), and Alveolar Ventilation ($\dot{V}_A$)

	Age (yr)					
	Newborn	1	5	12	15	Adult
V_T (mL)	20	78	130	260	360	500
f (bpm)	36	24	20	16	14	12
$\dot{V}_E$ (mL/min)	720	1872	2600	4160	5040	6000
V_D (mL)	7.5	21	49	105	141	150
$\dot{V}_A$ (mL/min)	450	1368	1620	2480	3066	4200

■ SPIROMETRY

Spirometry typically consists of a maximum inspiration to complete maximal voluntary lung expansion followed by maximal forced expiration, sustained until flow falls below 25 mL/s for at least one second or for as long as the patient can safely continue up to a timed endpoint, generally considered to be 15 s. In this setting, the total volume exhaled is called the forced vital capacity (FVC). When the patient exhales with less than maximal force for as long as can be safely tolerated, this is called the slow vital capacity (SVC). When the patient exhales as completely or for as long as possible, then inhales maximally, this is called the inspiratory vital capacity (IVC). The latter two methods are generally used for lung volume determinations and diffusing capacity tests, respectively. In individuals with normal lung function, the difference between any of these volumes is minimal, and the prediction equations for FVC can be used for SVC or IVC.

Vital Capacity (VC)

Volume change of the lungs measured on a complete expiration after a maximum inspiration or a complete inspiration after a maximum expiration. Prediction equations are shown in Table 2–4. Typical values are shown in Table 2–5.

Table 2-4 Prediction Equations for Vital Capacity

Infant (crying VC), (mL)	3.36 length (cm) − 104
Child < 8 yr, (mL)	1.63 height $(cm)^{2.87} \times 10^{-3}$
Male child (8-19 yr), (L)	−0.2584 − 0.20415 age + 0.010133 age^2 + 0.00018624 height $(cm)^2$
Female child (8-17 yr), (L)	−0.8710 + 0.06537 age + 0.00011496 height $(cm)^2$
Male adult (≥20 yr), (L)	48.1 height (cm) − 20.0 age − 2810
Female adult (≥18 yr), (L)	40.4 height (cm) − 22.0 age − 2350

Table 2-5 Typical Values for Vital Capacity

		Age (yr)					
	Newborn (mL)	1 (mL)	5 (L)	12 (L)	15 (L)	Adult male, (L)	Adult female, (L)
VC	100*	500	1.25	2.75	4.30	5.00	3.50

*Crying vital capacity (CVC).

Functional Residual Capacity (FRC)

The volume of gas remaining in the lungs at the end of relaxed (passive) expiration. Prediction equations are shown in Table 2–6. Typical values are shown in Table 2–7.

Table 2-6 Prediction Equations for Functional Residual Capacity

Infant (1-5 days)	FRC (mL) = 30 mL/kg
Small child (1 mo-5 yr)	FRC (mL) = 0.0157 length $(cm)^{2.238}$
Child (5-16 yr)	FRC (L) = [0.00088 height $(cm)^{2.91}] \times 10^{-3}$
Male adult	FRC (L) = 0.472 height (cm) + 0.009 age − 5.29
Female adult	FRC (L) = 0.036 height (cm) + 0.0031 age − 3.182

Table 2-7 Typical Values for Functional Residual Capacity

	Age (yr)				
	5	12	15	Adult (M)	Adult (F)
FRC (L)	0.7	1.90	2.80	3.00	2.75

Residual Volume (RV)

That volume of gas remaining in the lungs after maximum expiration. Prediction equations are shown in Table 2–8. Typical values are shown in Table 2–9.

Table 2-8 Prediction Equations for Residual Volume

Child (5-16 yr)	RV (L) = $[0.032$ height (cm)$^{2.04}] \times 10^{-3}$
Male adult	RV (L) = 0.0216 height (cm) + 0.0207 age $- 2.84$
Female adult	RV (L) = 0.0197 height (cm) + 0.0201 age $- 2.421$

Table 2-9 Typical Values for Residual Volume

	Age (yr)				
	5	12	15	Adult (M)	Adult (F)
RV (L)	0.40	0.90	1.10	1.50	1.20

Total Lung Capacity (TLC)

The volume of gas in the lung after maximum inspiration. Prediction equations are shown in Table 2–10. Typical values are shown in Table 2–11.

Table 2-10 Prediction Equations for Total Lung Capacity

Child (5-16 yr)	TLC (L) = $[0.003$ height (cm)$^{2.80}] \times 10^{-3}$
Male adult	TLC (L) = 0.0795 height (cm) + 0.0032 age -7.333
Female adult	TLC (L) = 0.059 height (cm) $- 4.537$

Table 2-11 Typical Values for Total Lung Capacity

	Age (yr)				
	5	12	15	Adult (M)	Adult (F)
TLC (L)	1.60	3.70	5.25	6.25	5.00

Residual Volume to Total Lung Capacity Ratio (RV/TLC)

The fraction of total lung capacity (TLC) that is taken up by residual volume (RV), expressed as a percent.

RV/TLC = 25% ± 5% in healthy individuals

Forced Vital Capacity (FVC)

A vital capacity performed with a maximum expiratory effort sustained until empty or a exhalation time of 15 s. Prediction equations are shown in Table 2–12.

Table 2-12 Prediction Equations for Forced Vital Capacity

Male child (8-19 yr), (L)	$-0.2584 - 0.20415 \, age + 0.010133 \, age^2 + 0.00018642$ height $(cm)^2$
Female child (8-17 yr), (L)	$-1.2082 + 0.05916 \, age + 0.00014815$ height $(cm)^2$
Male adult ($\geq$20 yr), (L)	$-0.1933 + 0.00064 \, age - 0.000269 \, age^2 + 0.00018642$ height $(cm)^2$
Female adult ($\geq$18 yr), (L)	$-0.3560 + 0.01870 \, age + 0.000382 \, age^2 + 0.00014815$ height $(cm)^2$

Forced Expiratory Volume in 1 Second (FEV$_1$)

The volume of gas exhaled in 1 second during the execution of a forced vital capacity. Prediction equations are shown in Table 2–13.

Table 2-13 Prediction Equations for Forced Expiratory Volume in 1 Second

Male child (8-19 yr), (L)	$-0.7453 - 0.04106 \, age + 0.004477 \, age^2 + 0.00014098$ height $(cm)^2$
Female child (8-17 yr), (L)	$-0.8710 + 0.06537 \, age + 0.00011496$ height $(cm)^2$
Male adult ($\geq$20 yr), (L)	$0.5536 - 0.01303 \, age - 0.000172 \, age^2 + 0.00014098$ height $(cm)^2$
Female adult ($\geq$18 yr), (L)	$0.4333 - 0.00361 \, age - 0.000194 \, age^2 + 0.00011496$ height $(cm)^2$

Forced Expiratory Volume-Forced Vital Capacity Ratio (FEV/FVC)

Forced expiratory volume (timed) to forced vital capacity ratio, expressed as a percentage. Prediction equations are shown in Table 2–14. Typical values for a healthy person, 25 years old are shown below:

$FEV_{0.5}$ sec = 60% of FVC

FEV_1 sec = 83% of FVC

FEV_2 sec = 94% of FVC

FEV_3 sec = 97% of FVC

Table 2-14 Prediction Equations for Mean Normal FEV$_1$/FVC Ratio (%)

Male, (%)	88.066 − 0.2066 age
Female, (%)	90.809 − 0.2125 age

Note: The FEV$_1$/FVC ratio is age dependent and declines with aging in adults. The predicted lower limit of normal is approximately 9%–10% below the mean predicted value.

Forced Expiratory Flow 25%-75% (FEF$_{25\%-75\%}$)

Mean forced expiratory flow during the middle half of the forced vital capacity. The 95% confidence interval for the FEF$_{25\%-75\%}$ has recently been shown to increase with age, making the practice of approximating the lower limit of normal for this parameter at 80% of the mean predicted value invalid. Prediction equations are shown in Table 2–15.

Table 2-15 Prediction Equations for Forced Expiratory Flow 25%-75%

Male child (8-19 yr), (L)	−1.0863 + 0.13939 age + 0.00010345 height (cm)^2
Female child (8-17 yr), (L)	−2.5284 + 0.52490 age − 0.015309 age^2 + 0.00006982 height (cm)^2
Male adult ($\geq$20 yr), (L)	2.7006 − 0.04995 age + 0.00010345 cm^2
Female adult ($\geq$18 yr), (L)	2.3670 − 0.01904 age − 0.0002 age^2 + 0.00006982 height (cm)^2

Peak Expiratory Flow (PEF)

The maximum flow recorded at any point during a forced expiratory maneuver. Prediction equations are shown in Table 2–16.

Table 2-16 Prediction Equations for Peak Expiratory Flow

Male (8-19), (L/min)	(−0.5962 − 0.12357 age + 0.013135 age^2 − 0.00024962 height (cm)^2) $\times$ 60
Female (8-17), (L/min)	(−3.6181 + 0.60644 age − 0.016846 age^2 − 0.00018623 height (cm)^2) $\times$ 60
Male ($\geq$20), (L/min)	(1.0523 + 0.08272 age − 0.001301 age^2 + 0.00024962 height (cm)^2) $\times$ 60
Female ($\geq$18), (L/min)	(0.9267 + 0.06929 age − 0.001031 age^2 + 0.00018623 height (cm)^2) $\times$ 60

Maximum Voluntary Ventilation (MVV)

The volume of air expired in 1 minute during repetitive maximum respiratory efforts, usually measured for 15 s and multiplied by 4. The ideal respiratory rate for measurement of MVV is typically 90 to 120 breaths/minute, but multiple efforts will show the ideal rate for any given patient. Maximum values for MVV in patients with airflow obstruction may be achieved at lower respiratory rates, depending on disease severity. The $FEV_1 \times 40$ will yield an approximate MVV for patients with airflow obstruction and normal inspiratory flows. Prediction equations are shown in Table 2–17.

Table 2-17 Prediction Equations for Maximum Voluntary Ventilation

Male child (L/min)	2.165 age + 1.076 height (cm) − 89.66
Female child (L/min)	2.725 age + 0.772 height (cm) − 57.84
Male adult (L/min)	1.193 height (cm) − 0.816 age − 37.9
Female adult (L/min)	0.8425 height (cm) − 0.685 age − 4.87

Airway Resistance (Raw)

An effective measure of the flow resistance of the airways obtained by plethysmographic techniques, presumed to be measured at FRC. Prediction equations are shown in Table 2–18.

Table 2-18 Prediction Equations for Airway Resistance

Infant (cm H_2O/L/sec)	mean value 19.2 ± 5.6
Child (cm H_2O/L/sec)	$3.87 \times 10^6 \times$ height (cm)$^{-2.67}$
Adult (cm H_2O/L/sec)	0.5 − 2.0

Airway Conductance (Gaw)

The reciprocal of airway resistance (1/Raw). Airway resistance and conductance both vary with thoracic gas volume (TGV). However, the relationship between Gaw and TGV is more nearly linear than the relationship between Raw and TGV. Prediction equations are shown in Table 2–19.

Table 2-19 Prediction Equations for Airway Conductance

Child (1-5 yr)	Gaw (L/sec/cm H_2O) = $0.143 \times$ TGV (L) − 0.644
Child (6-18 yr)	Gaw (L/sec/cm H_2O) = $10^{[2.6498 \log \text{height (cm)} - 6.2210]}$
Female adult	Gaw (L/sec/cm H_2O) = 0.29 TGV (L) − 0.27
Male adult	Gaw (L/sec/cm H_2O) = 0.28 TGV (L) − 0.73

Lung Compliance (C$_L$)

An effective measure of the elastic behavior of the lungs defined as the ratio of the change in lung volume to the change in transpulmonary pressure when there is no flow. Transpulmonary pressure is typically calculated using esophageal pressure as a surrogate for pleural pressure. Lung compliance is typically measured during passive exhalation from TLC to FRC with the segment from FRC to FRC + 0.5 L taken as a standardized portion of the pressure–volume curve to report as representing lung compliance. Prediction equations are shown in Table 2–20.

Table 2-20 Prediction Equations for Lung Compliance

Infant	C$_L$ (mL/cm H$_2$O) = 2.0 weight (kg)
Child	C$_L$ (L/cm H$_2$O) = 0.00102 $\times 10^{[2.0817 \times \log \text{height (cm)} - 2.3699]}$
Adult	C$_L$ (L/cm H$_2$O) = 0.05 FRC (L)

Carbon Monoxide Diffusing Capacity (DL$_{CO}$)

Amount of gas diffusing across the alveolar capillary membrane per unit of pressure difference per minute. Prediction equations are shown in Table 2–21.

Table 2-21 Prediction Equations for Carbon Monoxide Diffusing Capacity

Child (mL/min/mm Hg)	$2.986 \times 10^{[2.0867 \log \text{height (cm)} - 3.70145]}$
Male adult (mL/min/mm Hg)	0.164 height (cm) − 0.229 age + 12.9
Female adult (mL/min/mm Hg)	0.16 height (cm) − 0.111 age + 2.24

Maximum Inspiratory Pressure (P$_I$max)

The maximum inspiratory pressure that can be generated against an occlusion starting at or near residual volume. Prediction equations are shown in Table 2–22.

Table 2-22 Prediction Equations for Maximum Inspiratory Pressure

Male (6-60 yr)	P$_I$max (cm H$_2$O) = 143 − 0.55 age
Female (6-60 yr)	P$_I$max (cm H$_2$O) = 104 − 0.51 age

Maximum Expiratory Pressure (P$_E$max)

The maximum expiratory pressure that can be generated against an occlusion starting at or near total lung capacity. Prediction equations are shown in Table 2–23.

Table 2-23 Prediction Equations for Maximum Expiratory Pressure

Male (6-60 yr)	PEmax (cm H_2O) = 268 − 1.03 age
Female (6-60 yr)	PEmax (cm H_2O) = 170 − 0.53 age

Tables 2–24, 2–25, and 2–26 show typical patterns of pulmonary function test as well as values used to assess the severity of the defects.

Table 2-24 Summary of Pulmonary Function Profile in Obstructive and Restrictive Diseases[*]

	Obstruction	Restriction
VC	→ to ↓ (when severe)	↓ to ↓↓
FEV_1	↓ to ↓↓	↓ to ↓↓
FEV_1/FVC	↓ to ↓↓	→ to ↑
TLC	→ to ↑	↓ to ↓↓
FRC	↑ to ↑↑↑	→ to ↓
RV	↑ to ↑↑↑	→ to ↓
RV/TLC	↑ to ↑↑↑	→ to ↑
MVV	↓ to ↓↓	→ to ↓
$FEF_{25\%-75\%}$	↓ to ↓↓	→ to ↓

[*]→ = normal; ↑ = increased; ↓ = decreased. Typically, restriction means ↓ VC and TLC; normal flow rates; obstruction means ↓ VC and flow rates; normal or increased TLC.

Table 2-25 Assessment of Severity for Obstructive and Restrictive Pulmonary Diseases[*]

	FEV_1, Percentage of Predicted
Mild	>70
Moderate	60-69
Moderately severe	50-59
Severe	35-49
Very severe	<35

[*]Note: The presence of a restrictive ventilatory disorder should be confirmed by measurement of lung volumes. The sensitivity of a reduced FVC for restriction (confirmed by a reduced TLC on lung volumes) is approximately 60%.

Table 2-26 General Risk of Developing Postoperative Pulmonary Complications in Patients With Abnormal Pulmonary Function

	Low Risk	Moderate Risk	High Risk
VC (%pred)	>60	40-60	<40
FEV$_1$/FVC (%)	>55	40-55	<40
MVV (%pred)	>60	40-60	<40
PaCO$_2$ (mm Hg)	<45	45-50	>50
PaO$_2$ (mm Hg room air)	>60	40-60	<40

■ BRONCHIAL INHALATION CHALLENGES

Pharmacologic agents are used to identify patients with suspected airway hyperreactivity. Table 2–27 shows the dosing schedule approved by the FDA for administering a methacholine challenge test. The minimum change in baseline FEV$_1$ or sGaw for a positive study is shown in Table 2–28.

Table 2-27 FDA-Approved Dosing Schedule for Methacholine Challenge*

Methacholine Concentration (mg/mL)	Number of Breaths
0.025	5
0.25	5
2.5	5
10.0	5
25.0	5

*Five breaths at each dose, with a 0.6-s nebulization burst at FRC and a 5- to 10-s breathhold for each breath.

Table 2-28 Significant Spirometry Changes Following Bronchial Challenge

Test	Minimum Change From Baseline (%)
FEV$_1$	−20
sGaw (specific Gaw)	−40

Methacholine Results: The provocative concentration of methacholine solution that caused a 20% fall in FEV$_1$ from baseline (PC20FEV$_1$) is calculated by interpolation when the last dose caused a greater than 20% fall. Table 2–29 shows a scheme for categorizing the PC20FEV$_1$.

Table 2-29 Categorization of Bronchial Responsiveness[*]

PC20FEV$_1$ (mg/mL)	Interpretation
>16.0	Normal bronchial responsiveness
4.0-16.0	Borderline bronchial hyperresponsiveness (BHR)
1.0-4.0	Mild BHR (positive test)
<1.0	Moderate to severe BHR

[*]Caveats: assumes baseline airflow obstruction is absent, spirometry quality is good, and there is a substantial post-challenge FEV$_1$ recovery.

■ EXERCISE PHYSIOLOGY

Resting Energy Expenditure (REE)

The minimum level of energy required to sustain the body's vital functions in a resting state. Prediction equations are shown in Table 2–30. Average rates of energy expenditure appear in Table 2–31.

Table 2-30 Prediction Equations for Resting Energy Expenditure

Male adult	REE = 66.5 + 13.8 weight (kg) + 5.0 height (cm) − 6.8 age
Female adult	REE = 66.5 + 96 weight (kg) + 1.8 height (cm) − 4.7 age

Table 2-31 Average Rates of Energy Expenditure for Men and Women Living in the United States

	Age	Weight	Height	Energy Expenditure
Men	15-18	61	172	3000
	19-22	67	172	3000
	23-50	70	172	2700
	>50	70	172	2400
Women	15-18	54	162	2100
	19-22	58	162	2100
	23-50	58	162	2000
	>50	58	162	1800

Maximum Oxygen Consumption ($\dot{V}O_2$max)

The highest oxygen consumption that an individual can obtain during physical work; a measure of fitness. Technically, most cardiopulmonary stress tests result in a measurement of $\dot{V}O_2$peak. A true $\dot{V}O_2$max is measured when the oxygen uptake demonstrates a plateau in the face of an increasing workload. Prediction equations and normal values are shown in Table 2–32. Oxygen consumption varies with activity (Table 2–33) and underlying disease (Table 2–34).

Table 2-32 Prediction Equations for

Maximum Oxygen Consumption ($\dot{V}O_2$max)	
Male adult	4.2 − 0.032 age
Female adult	2.6 − 0.016 age

Normal Values for $\dot{V}O_2$max in Adults

Male child (≤13 yr)	(42 mL/min)/kg
Male child (>13 yr)	(50 mL/min)/kg
Female child (=11 yr)	(38 mL/min)/kg
Female child (>11 yr)	(34 mL/min)/kg

Table 2-33 $\dot{V}O_2$ Requirements of Common Activities

Activity	$\dot{V}O_2$ (mL/min)/kg
Desk work	4-7
Driving car	4-7
Level walking (1 mph)	4-7
Sweeping floors	7-11
Making beds	7-11
Automobile repair	7-11
Wheelbarrow (100-lb load)	11-14
Bicycling (6 mph)	11-14
Golfing (pulling cart)	11-14
Tennis (doubles)	14-18
Painting masonry	14-18
Golf (carrying clubs)	14-18
Digging garden	18-21
Cycling (10 mph)	18-21

Table 2-34 Patterns of Response to Exercise

	Cardiac Disease	Obstructive Lung Disease	Interstitial Lung Disease	Deconditioned
V̇O₂max	↓	↓↓	↓↓	↓
V̇E/MVV	—	↑	↑	—
HRmax (%pred)	>95%	Variable; low when severe	80%	>95%
O₂ pulse (max)	↓	↓↓	↓↓	↓
VD/VT	—	↑	↑	—
AT	↓	↓ (likely to be absent when severe)	↓↓	—
PaO₂	—	↓	↓↓	—

— = Within normal range; ↓ = mild change; ↓↓ = marked change.

Maximum Heart Rate (HRmax)

The highest heart rate attained during maximum exercise. Prediction equations are shown in Table 2–35.

Table 2-35 Prediction Equations for Maximum Heart Rate

Child	HRmax (bpm) = 195 $\pm$ 13
Adult	HRmax (bpm) = 220 $-$ age

Heart Rate Reserve (HRR)

The difference between the predicted maximum heart rate and the actual maximum exercise heart rate. The calculation of maximum heart rate reserve is

$$HRR = \text{predicted HRmax} - \text{observed HRmax}.$$

Maximum Oxygen Pulse (MOP)

The quotient of predicted maximum oxygen consumption and predicted maximum heart rate. The maximum oxygen pulse is generally a reflection of the stroke volume. The prediction equation for maximum oxygen pulse is

$$\text{MOP (mL/beat)} = \frac{\text{predicted V}o_2\text{max (mL/min)}}{\text{predicted HRmax (mL/min)}}$$

SUGGESTED READING

American Thoracic Society/European Respiratory Society Task Force. Standardisation of lung function testing: Interpretive strategies for lung function testing. *Eur Respir J* 26 (2005), 948–968.

Hankinson, J. L., Odencrantz, J. R., and Fedan, K. B. Spirometric reference values from a sample of the general U.S. population. *Am J Respir Crit Care Med* 159:1 (January 1999), 179–187

Cotes, J. E. *Lung Function: Assessment and Application in Medicine.* Oxford: Blackwell Scientific Publications, 1993.

American Thoracic Society: Guidelines for Pulmonary Function Testing. Downloads available from: http://www.thoracic.org/sections/publications/statements/index.html.

Hughes, J. M. and Pride, N. B. *Lung Function Tests: Physiological Principles and Clinical Application*, 5th ed. London: Balliere Tindall, 1999.

Wasserman, K., Hansen, J., Sue, D., Stringer, W., and Whipp, B. *Principles of Exercise Testing and Interpretation: Including Pathophysiology and Clinical Applications*, 4th ed. Philadelphia: Lippincott, Williams and Wilkins, 2004.

3

Physiologic Monitoring

■ GAS EXCHANGE

The equations in this section express the relationships that exist during gas exchange in the steady state. They are based on the following two assumptions:

1. that there is no carbon dioxide in the inspired gas, and
2. that the net exchange of nitrogen is negligible because of its very low solubility.

All fractional gas concentrations are calculated on a dry gas basis.

Oxygen Uptake

The rate at which oxygen is removed from alveolar gas by the blood. Under steady-state conditions, oxygen uptake equals oxygen consumption (the rate at which oxygen is metabolized). See oxygen consumption on page 92.

Abbreviation: $\dot{V}O_2$

Units: mL/min (STPD)

Normal value: 240 mL/min (adults) or

100–180 mL/min/m^2 (children or adults)

6–8 mL/min/kg (infants)

Equation for $FIO_2 < 1.0$:

$$\dot{V}O_2 = \dot{V}E \left[FIO_2 \left(\frac{1 - F\bar{E}CO_2 - F\bar{E}O_2}{1 - FIO_2} \right) - F\bar{E}O_2 \right]$$

Equation for $FIO_2 = 1.0$:

$$\dot{V}O_2 = \dot{V}E \left(FIO_2 - F\bar{E}O_2 \right)$$

where

$\dot{V}E$ = exhaled minute volume (mL/min STPD)

FIO_2 = fraction of oxygen in inspired gas

$F\bar{E}O_2$ = fraction of oxygen in mixed exhaled gas

$F\bar{E}CO_2$ = fraction of carbon dioxide in mixed exhaled gas

Carbon Dioxide Output

Carbon dioxide output is a function of the amount of that gas produced by metabolism and the level of alveolar ventilation. The equation relating these variables may also be solved for alveolar ventilation.

Abbreviation: $\dot{V}_{CO_2}$

Units: mL/min (STPD)

Normal value: 192 mL/min (adults) or

$\qquad$ 80–144 mL/min/m^2 (children and adults)

$\qquad$ 5–6 mL/kg/min (infants)

Equation:

$$\dot{V}_{CO_2} = \dot{V}_E \times F\bar{E}_{CO_2}$$

$$\dot{V}_{CO_2} = \frac{\dot{V}_A \times P_{A_{CO_2}}}{P_B - P_{A_{H_2O}}}$$

$$\dot{V}_A = \frac{\dot{V}_{CO_2}(P_B - P_{A_{H_2O}})}{P_{A_{CO_2}}} = \frac{R_E(P_B - P_{A_{H_2O}})\dot{V}_{O_2}}{P_{A_{CO_2}}}$$

where

$\dot{V}_E$ = exhaled minute volume (mL/min STPD)

$F\bar{E}_{CO_2}$ = fraction of carbon dioxide in mixed exhaled gas

$\dot{V}_A$ = alveolar ventilation (mL/min STPD)

$P_{A_{CO_2}}$ = partial pressure of alveolar carbon dioxide (mm Hg). This value is often assumed to be equal to arterial carbon dioxide tension ($P_{a_{CO_2}}$)

R_E = respiratory exchange ratio

P_B = barometric pressure (mm Hg)

$P_{A_{H_2O}}$ = partial pressure of water in alveolar gas (mm Hg). This value is 47 mm Hg for gas saturated with water vapor at 37°C.

During rebreathing experiments or when individuals are confined to an enclosed area, the carbon dioxide concentration rises in proportion to the rate of carbon dioxide production. The time required to reach a given carbon dioxide concentration (% CO_2) is given by

$$t = \frac{\% \ CO_2 \times V}{\dot{V}_{CO_2} \times 100 \times N}$$

where

t = time

% CO_2 = ambient CO_2 level (%)

V = volume of enclosure

$\dot{V}CO_2$ = CO_2 production rate

N = number of individuals

For example, at one time the standard for ambient carbon dioxide levels aboard Navy submarines was 3%. $\dot{V}CO_2$ was estimated at 0.75 ft^3/h so that the above equation reduced to t(hours) = 0.04 V/N.

Alveolar Carbon Dioxide Equation

Alveolar partial pressure of carbon dioxide is directly proportional to the amount of carbon dioxide produced by metabolism and delivered to the lungs and inversely proportional to the alveolar ventilation. Alveolar and arterial Pco_2 can be assumed to be equal.

Abbreviation: $PACO_2$

Units: mmHg

Normal value: 35–45 mm Hg

Equation:

$$PACO_2 = \frac{0.863 \times \dot{V}CO_2}{\dot{V}E \times \left(1 - \frac{V_D}{V_T}\right)}$$

where

$\dot{V}CO_2$ = carbon dioxide output

$\dot{V}E$ = exhaled minute ventilation

V_D/V_T = Dead space ratio

Respiratory Quotient

The molar ratio of carbon dioxide production to oxygen consumption. This ratio depends on the type of substrate being metabolized. For glucose, the respiratory quotient equals 1.0 (i.e., $C_6H_{12}O_2 + 6\ O_2 \rightarrow 6\ COCO_2 + 6\ H_2O$). For fat RQ is approximately 0.7, and for protein RQ is about 0.8. Under steady-state conditions, a mixture of glucose, fat, and protein is metabolized to produce a respiratory quotient of 0.8–0.85.

Abbreviation: RQ

Units: dimensionless

Normal value: 0.80–0.85

Respiratory Exchange Ratio

The ratio of carbon dioxide output to oxygen uptake as determined by the analysis of mixed exhaled gas.

Abbreviation: R_E

Units: dimensionless

Normal value: 0.8

Equations:

$$R_E = \frac{\dot{V}_{CO_2}}{\dot{V}_{O_2}}$$

$$R_E = \frac{F\bar{E}_{CO_2}}{F_{IO_2}\left(\dfrac{1 - F\bar{E}_{CO_2} - F\bar{E}_{O_2}}{1 - F_{IO_2}}\right) - F\bar{E}_{O_2}}$$

where

$\dot{V}_{CO_2}$ = carbon dioxide output

$\dot{V}_{O_2}$ = oxygen uptake

$F\bar{E}_{CO_2}$ = fraction of carbon dioxide in mixed exhaled gas

F_{IO_2} = fraction of inspired oxygen

$F\bar{E}_{O_2}$ = fraction of oxygen in mixed exhaled gas

Partial Pressure of Inspired Oxygen

The dry gas pressure of oxygen in inspired air.

Abbreviation: P_{IO_2}

Units: mm Hg (torr)

Equation:

$$P_{IO_2} = (P_B - P_{IH_2O})F_{IO_2}$$

where

P_B = barometric pressure (mm Hg)

P_{IH_2O} = partial pressure (mm Hg) of water in inspired gas (This value is 47 mm Hg for gas saturated with water vapor at 37°C.)

F_{IO_2} = fraction of oxygen in inspired gas

Note: To calculate P_{IO_2} during mechanical ventilation, mean airway pressure (in mm Hg) should be added to barometric pressure.

Tables 3–1 and 3–2 along with Figures 3–1 through 3–4 show various measurements of partial pressure as well as the effects of altitude on such measurements.

Table 3-1 Effect of Altitude on Inspired Oxygen Tension

Altitude		Barometric Pressure		Inspired Oxygen Tension		Equivalent F_{IO_2}*
(ft)	(m)	(torr)	(kPa)	(torr)	(kPa)	
0	0	760	101	149	20	0.21
1,000	305	733	97	143	19	0.2
2,000	610	707	94	138	18	0.19
3,000	914	681	91	133	18	0.19
4,000	1,219	656	87	127	17	0.18
5,000	1,524	632	84	122	16	0.17
6,000	1,829	609	81	117	16	0.16
8,000	2,438	564	75	108	14	0.15
10,000	3,048	523	70	99	13	0.14
12,000	3,658	483	64	91	12	0.13
14,000	4,267	446	59	83	11	0.12
16,000	4,877	412	55	76	10	0.11
18,000	5,486	379	50	69	9	0.10
20,000	6,096	349	46	63	8	0.09
22,000	6,706	321	43	57	8	0.08
24,000	7,315	294	39	52	7	0.07
26,000	7,925	270	36	47	6	0.07
28,000	8,534	247	33	42	6	0.06
30,000	9,144	226	30	37	5	0.05

*F_{IO_2} at sea level, which would produce the same inspired oxygen tension.

Table 3-2 Comparison of Blood-Gas Values at Altitude and at Sea Level

	Sea Level	Denver 1609 m	Mt Everest 8400 m
pH	7.35-7.45	7.3.5-7.45	7.45-7.60
P_{CO_2}, mm Hg	35-45	34-38	10.3-15.7
P_{O_2}, mm Hg	80-100	65-75	19.1-29.5
S_{O_2}, %	>95	92-94	34-69.7
HCO_3^-, mEq/L	22-26	22-26	9.9-12
BE, mEq/L	−2-+2	−2-+2	−5.7-−9.2

Data from Grocott, M. P. W. et al. *NEJM* 360 (2009), 140-149.

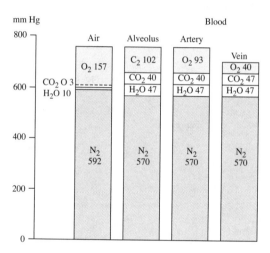

Figure 3-1 Partial pressures of gas in air at sea level (BP = mm Hg).

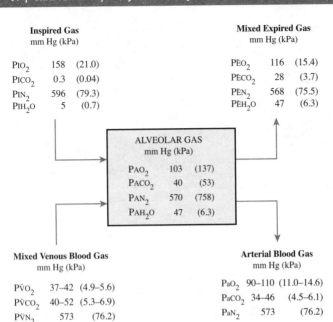

Figure 3-2 Normal partial pressures of respired gases.

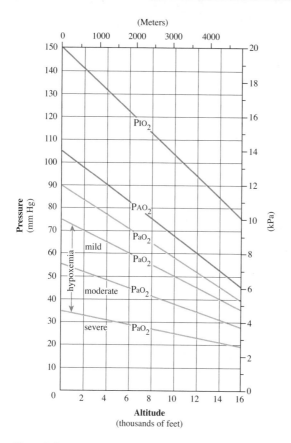

Figure 3-3 The effect of altitute on inspired, alveolar, and arterial oxygen tension ($FIO_2 = 0.21$).

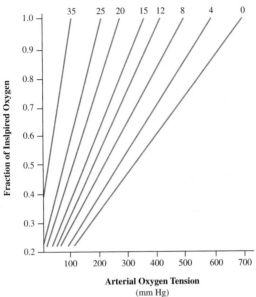

Altitude
(thousands of feet above sea level)

Figure 3-4 The effect of altitude on Pao$_2$ during oxygen administration.

Alveolar Oxygen Tension

The following equation represents the mean alveolar oxygen tension. Figure 3–5 illustrates a nomogram for the equation.

Abbreviation: PAO$_2$

Units: mm Hg (torr)

Normal value (room air): 102 at sea level

Equation:

$$PAO_2 = PIO_2 - PACO_2\left[FIO_2 + \left(\frac{1 - FIO_2}{RE}\right)\right]$$

$$\approx PIO_2 - \frac{PACO_2}{RE}$$

where

PIO_2 = partial pressure of oxygen in inspired gas (mm Hg)

$PACO_2$ = partial pressure (mm Hg) of carbon dioxide in alveolar gas (this value is often assumed to be equal to arterial carbon dioxide tension [$PACO_2$])

FIO_2 = fraction of oxygen in inspired gas

RE = respiratory exchange ratio

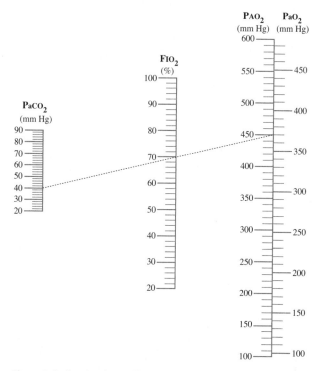

Figure 3-5 Alveolar air equation nomogram (assuming sea level and R = 0.8 and virtual shunt of 5%). A straight line connecting $PaCO_2$ and FIO_2 will intersect the resulting PAO_2 and the predicted PaO_2. For example, a $PaCO_2$ of 40 mm Hg and an FIO_2 of 70% will result in a PAO_2 of approximately 450 mm Hg and a predicted PaO_2 of about 370 mm Hg.

Arterial-Alveolar Oxygen Tension Ratio

An index of gas exchange function that has been shown to be more stable than the alveolar–arterial oxygen tension gradient with changing values of inspired oxygen concentration. It is most stable when it is less than 0.55, the F_{IO_2} is greater than 0.30, and the PaO_2 is less than 100 mm Hg. (For graphs related to this ratio, see Figures 3–6 and 3–7.)

Abbreviation: $P(a/A)O_2$

Units: dimensionless

Normal value: 0.74–0.82 (lower limits of normal for men)

Equation:

$$P(a/A)O_2 = \frac{PaO_2}{P_{IO_2} - PaCO_2\left[F_{IO_2} + \left(\frac{1 - F_{IO_2}}{RE}\right)\right]}$$

$$P(a/A)O_2 \approx \frac{PaO_2}{P_{IO_2} - \dfrac{PaCO_2}{RE}}$$

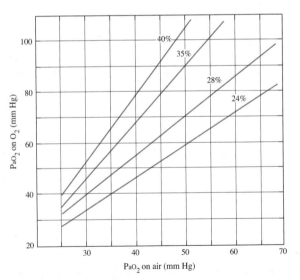

Figure 3-6 Graph relating the expected PaO_2 during oxygen administration based on the measured PaO_2 on room air.

where

Pa_{O_2} = partial pressure of oxygen in arterial blood (mm Hg)

P_{IO_2} = partial pressure of oxygen in inspired gas (mm Hg)

PA_{CO_2} = partial pressure of carbon dioxide in alveolar gas (mm Hg); this value is often assumed to be equal to Pa_{CO_2}

Pa_{CO_2} = partial pressure of carbon dioxide in arterial blood

F_{IO_2} = fraction of oxygen in inspired gas

R_E = respiratory exchange ratio

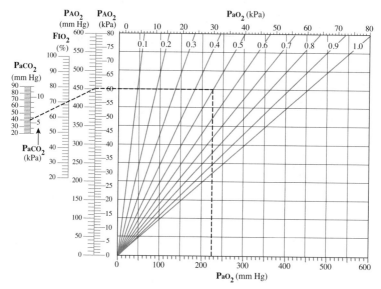

Figure 3–7 Arterial to alveolar oxygen tension ratio nomogram. A straight line connecting Pa_{CO_2} and F_{IO_2} will intersect the resulting PA_{O_2}. The arterial-alveolar ratio is represented by the diagonal line connecting the origin of the graph (PA_{O_2} = 0, Pa_{O_2} = 0) and the point representing the given PA_{O_2} and Pa_{O_2}. For example, a Pa_{CO_2} of 40 mm Hg and an F_{IO_2} of 70% result in a PA_{O_2} of about 450 mm Hg. If the measured Pa_{O_2} is 225 mm Hg, the $P(a/A)_{O_2}$ ratio is 0.5.

Prediction Equation for Normal P(a/A)O₂ While Breathing Room Air:

$$Sitting: \mathrm{P(a/A)O_2} = 0.9333 - 0.0026 \text{ age (yr)}$$

$$Supine: \mathrm{P(a/A)O_2} = 0.9333 - 0.00406 \text{ age (yr)}$$

The patient's current $\mathrm{P(a/A)O_2}$ may be used to estimate the $\mathrm{FIO_2}$ required to obtain a desired $\mathrm{PaO_2}$ using the equation:

$$\mathrm{FIO_{2needed}} = \frac{\left(\dfrac{\mathrm{PaO_{2\ desired}}}{\mathrm{P(a/A)O_2}}\right) + \mathrm{PaCO_{2\ desired}}}{\mathrm{P_B} - 47}$$

where

$\mathrm{P_B}$ = barometric pressure in mm Hg

Alveolar–Arterial Oxygen Tension Gradient

This method of estimating the degree of intrapulmonary shunting assumes that the arterial oxygen tension is greater than 150 mm Hg. The results of this calculation are limited to giving only a qualitative estimate of the degree of shunting and will vary with changes in the inspired oxygen concentration and cardiovascular status. The alveolar–arterial oxygen gradient increases with age mainly due to progressing $\dot{V}/\dot{Q}$ mismatch.

Abbreviation: $\mathrm{P(A{-}a)O_2}$
Units: mm Hg
Normal value: 7–14 (while breathing 21% $\mathrm{O_2}$)

Equation:

$$\mathrm{P(A{-}a)O_2} = \mathrm{PIO_2} - \mathrm{PaCO_2}\left[\mathrm{FIO_2} + \left(\frac{1 - \mathrm{FIO_2}}{\mathrm{R_E}}\right)\right] - \mathrm{PaO_2}$$

$$\mathrm{P(A{-}a)O_2} \approx \mathrm{PIO_2} - \frac{\mathrm{PaCO_2}}{\mathrm{R_E}} - \mathrm{PaO_2}$$

where

$\mathrm{PIO_2}$ = partial pressure of oxygen in inspired gas (mm Hg)
$\mathrm{PaCO_2}$ = partial pressure (mm Hg) of carbon dioxide in alveolar gas (this value is often assumed to be equal to $\mathrm{PaCO_2}$)

Pa_{CO_2} = partial pressure of oxygen in arterial blood (mm Hg)

F_{IO_2} = fraction of oxygen in inspired gas

R_E = respiratory exchange ratio

Note: Another estimate of shunt can be derived by assuming a value for ideal alveolar–arterial equilibration while breathing 100% oxygen. Under these conditions, arterial oxygen tension (using normal values) can be expressed as

$$Pa_{O_2} = PA_{O_2} = PB - (47 + Pa_{CO_2}) \approx 673 \text{ mm Hg}$$

Any reduction in actual arterial oxygen tension from the theoretical value represents venous-to-arterial shunting. For practical purposes, each 100 mm Hg reduction in actual PA_{O_2} below the theoretical Pa_{O_2} represents a 5% shunt. The clinical equation is thus

$$\% \text{ shunt} \approx \frac{673 - Pa_{O_2}}{20}$$

Prediction Equations for Normal $P(A-a)O_2$ While Breathing Room Air:

Sitting: $P(A-a)O_2 = 0.27$ age (yr)

Supine: $P(A-a)O_2 = 0.42$ age (yr)

Tables 3–3, 3–4, and 3–5 show equations and ranges to characterize the severity of oxygenation impairment.

Table 3-3 Prediction Equations for Determining Oxygenation Impairment for Sitting Subjects

Impairment	Pa_{O_2} (mm Hg)	$P(A-a)O_2$ (mm Hg)	$P(a/A)O_2$ (Dimensionless)
Normal	$\geq 97.2 - 0.27$ age*	$\leq 7 + 0.27$ age*	$\geq 0.933 - 0.0026$ age**
Mild	$\geq 83.2 - 0.27$ age*	$\leq 21 + 0.27$ age*	$\geq 0.798 - 0.0026$ age**
Moderate	$\geq 69.2 - 0.27$ age*	$\leq 35 + 0.27$ age*	$\geq 0.664 - 0.0026$ age**
Severe	$\geq 55.2 - 0.27$ age*	$\leq 49 + 0.27$ age*	$\geq 0.482 - 0.0026$ age**
Extreme	$< 55.2 - 0.27$ age*	$> 49 + 0.27$ age*	$< 0.482 - 0.0026$ age**

*Age in years; for supine posture, change age coefficient to 0.42.
**Age in years; for supine posture, change age coefficient to 0.00406.

Table 3-4 Assessment of Hypoxemia in Adults and Children[*]

	Pao$_2$ (mm Hg)
Normal	97
Acceptable	>80
Mild hypoxemia	<80
Moderate hypoxemia	<60
Severe hypoxemia	<40

[*]Sea level, 21% oxygen.

Table 3-5 Assessment of Hypoxemia in Newborn and Elderly Patients[*]

Age (yr)	Acceptable Range of Pao$_2$
Newborn	40-70
60	>80
70	>70
80	>60
90	>50

[*]Limits of hypoxemia for elderly patients are determined by subtracting 1 mm Hg for each year over 60.
Normal: Pao$_2$ ≈ 102 − 0.33 × age (yr)

Oxygenation Ratio

The ratio of arterial oxygen tension to the fraction of inspired oxygen (where F$_{IO_2}$ is expressed as a decimal, 30% = 0.3). A ratio of 200 or less correlates with a shunt fraction of 20% or more but is generally a crude indicator of shunt. This ratio is easier to calculate than either the P$_{(A–a)O_2}$ or the P$_{(a/A)O_2}$, but is subject to variability due to differing values of arterial carbon dioxide tension.

Abbreviation: Pao$_2$/F$_{IO_2}$
Units: dimensionless
Normal value: 350–470

Oxygenation Index

An index of oxygenation status often used to assess infants before treatment with extracorporeal membrane oxygenation (ECMO). In these patients, an index value of >35 for 5–6 hours is one criterion for ECMO. The value of the oxygenation index correlates with mortality in pediatric acute respiratory failure.

Abbreviation: OI
Units: cm H_2O/mm Hg
Normal Value: 0

Equation:

$$OI = \frac{\overline{Paw} \times F_{IO_2}}{Pa_{O_2}} \times 100$$

where

$\overline{Paw}$ = mean airway pressure (cm H_2O)
F_{IO_2} = fraction of inspired oxygen (as decimal)
Pa_{O_2} = arterial oxygen tension (mm Hg)

Physiologic Dead Space (Bohr Equation)

The volume of inspired gas that is not effective in arterializing the venous blood. The three main reasons for its ineffectiveness are (1) it never reached alveoli, (2) it reached alveoli with no perfusion, or (3) too much gas reached the alveoli in proportion to their perfusion. Physiologic dead space is often expressed as a ratio of dead space volume to tidal volume (V_D/V_T). Figure 3–8 shows the correlation between minute ventilation and carbon dioxide at different values of physiologic dead space.

Abbreviation: V_D
Units: mL (BTPS)
Normal value: $V_T = 2.2$ mL/kg ideal body weight
$V_D/V_T = 0.20$–0.40

Equation:

$$V_D = \frac{Pa_{CO_2} - P\overline{E}_{CO_2}}{Pa_{CO_2}} \times V_T$$

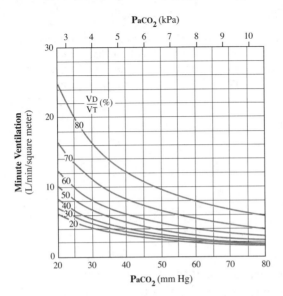

Figure 3-8 Graph relating minute ventilation and P_{aCO_2} for different values of physiologic dead space (assuming P_B = 760 mm Hg, 37°C, and carbon dioxide output of 112 mL/min/m²).

where

V_T = tidal volume (mL BTPS)

P_{ACO_2} = partial pressure (mm Hg) of carbon dioxide in alveolar gas (this value is often assumed to be equal to arterial carbon dioxide tension [P_{aCO_2}])

$P\bar{E}_{CO_2}$ = partial pressure of carbon dioxide in mixed exhaled gas (mm Hg)

Prediction Equation:

$$\frac{V_D}{V_T} = \frac{\text{actual } \dot{V}_E}{\text{pred } \dot{V}_E} \times \frac{P_{aCO_2}}{40} \times 0.33$$

where

pred = minute ventilation predicted from Radford nomogram

P_{aCO_2} = arterial carbon dioxide tension (mm Hg)

Clinical Calculation of Dead Space

Classically, to calculate dead space requires collection of exhaled gas to measure the partial pressure of carbon dioxide. This is technically difficult in daily practice, although there are devices that can obtain approximations based on volume exhaled and the curve obtained from the end tidal carbon dioxide, this is also not widely available. Recently Frankenfield et al. (*Crit Care Med* 38 (2010), 288–329) described and validated an equation to obtain the dead space ratio from clinically available data.

Abbreviation: V_D/V_T

Units: dimensionless

Normal value: $V_D/V_T = 0.20–0.40$

Equation:

$$\frac{V_D}{V_T} = 0.32 + 0.0106(Pa_{CO_2} - ET_{CO_2}) + 0.003(RR) + 0.0015(age)$$

where

Pa_{CO_2} = arterial carbon dioxide tension (mm Hg)

ET_{CO_2} = exhaled end tidal carbon dioxide (mm Hg)

RR = respiratory rate (breaths per minute)

Age = age of patient (years)

Oxygen Content of Blood

The following equations give the total quantity of oxygen in the blood. This includes the quantity of oxygen dissolved in the plasma plus the quantity of oxygen bound to the hemoglobin.

Abbreviations: Ca_{O_2} (arterial oxygen content)

$C\bar{v}_{O_2}$ (mixed venous oxygen content)

Cc'_{O_2} (pulmonary end capillary oxygen content)

Units: vol% (mL O_2/dL blood)

Normal value: $Ca_{O_2} = 20$; $C\bar{v}_{O_2} = 15$

Equations:

$$Ca_{O_2} = (Hb \times 1.34 \times O_2\text{sat}) + (0.0031 \times Pa_{O_2})$$

$$C\overline{v}_{O_2} = (Hb \times 1.34 \times O_2\text{sat}) + (0.0031 \times P\overline{v}_{O_2})$$

$$Cc'_{O_2} = (Hb \times 1.34 \times O_2\text{sat}) + (0.0031 \times Pc'_{O_2})$$

where

- Hb = hemoglobin content in g % (g Hb/dL blood) (normal value = 15 g %)
- 1.34 = a constant describing the amount of oxygen (mL at STPD) that can be carried by 1 g Hb when it is fully saturated (some authorities use 1.39 or 1.36)
- O_2sat = hemoglobin saturation expressed in decimal form. This value is assumed to be 1.0 when the oxygen tension of the blood is above 150 mm Hg.
- 0.0031 = a constant derived using the Bunsen solubility coefficient of oxygen in blood (i.e., for each 100 mL of blood, 0.0031 mL of oxygen can be dissolved for each mm Hg of oxygen tension on the blood)
- Pa_{O_2} = partial pressure of oxygen in arterial blood (mm Hg)
- $P\overline{v}_{O_2}$ = partial pressure of oxygen in mixed venous blood (mm Hg)
- Pc'_{O_2} = partial pressure of oxygen in end-pulmonary capillary blood (mm Hg) (often assumed to be equal to the partial pressure of oxygen in alveolar gas (PA_{O_2}))

Note: The pulmonary end capillary oxygen content reflects the maximal oxygen carrying capacity, where the oxygen saturation is assumed to be 100%.

Arteriovenous Oxygen Content Difference

The difference between the arterial and venous oxygen content is an indication of the amount of oxygen the body is consuming. It is also used as an indication of cardiac output. That is, if the metabolic demands of the body are assumed to be constant, a decrease in cardiac output will cause an increase in arteriovenous oxygen difference.

Abbreviation: $C(a-\overline{v})O_2$
Units: vol% (mL O_2 per dL blood)

Normal value: 4.5–6.0 (children and adults)

2.5–4.5 (patients that are critically ill but stable)

Equation:

$$C(a - \bar{v})O_2 = CaO_2 - C\bar{v}O_2$$

where

CaO_2 = arterial oxygen content (mL/dL)

$C\bar{v}O_2$ = mixed venous oxygen content (mL/dL)

Ventilation-Perfusion Ratio

This equation relates the factors that determine the adequacy of alveolar ventilation. It assumes that arterial and mixed venous blood gas samples are drawn simultaneously. This should be done midway through the expired gas collection if R_E is being calculated.

Abbreviation: $\dot{V}/\dot{Q}$

Units: dimensionless

Normal value: 0.8

Equation:

$$\dot{V}_A/\dot{Q}_C = \frac{R_E(P_B - P_{AH_2O})(CaO_2 - C\bar{v}O_2)}{P_{ACO_2} \times 100}$$

where

$\dot{V}_A$ = alveolar ventilation

$\dot{Q}_C$ = pulmonary blood flow

R_E = respiratory exchange ratio

P_B = barometric pressure (mm Hg)

P_{AH_2O} = partial pressure (mm Hg) of water in alveolar gas (this value is 47 mm Hg for gas saturated with water vapor at 37°C)

CaO_2 = arterial oxygen content (mL/dL)

$C\bar{v}O_2$ = mixed venous oxygen content (mL/dL)

P_{ACO_2} = partial pressure (mm Hg) of alveolar carbon dioxide (this value is often assumed to be equal to arterial CO_2 tension [P_{aCO_2}])

Venous-to-Arterial Shunt (Classic Form)

The collection of data for the shunt calculation is usually done with the patient placed supine while breathing 100% oxygen.

Abbreviation: $\dot{Q}s/\dot{Q}T$

Units: %

Normal value: 2–5 (children and adults)

Equation:

$$\frac{\dot{Q}s}{\dot{Q}T} = \frac{Cc'O_2 - CaO_2}{Cc'O_2 - C\bar{v}O_2}$$

where

$\dot{Q}s$ = shunted portion of cardiac output

$\dot{Q}T$ = total cardiac output

$Cc'O_2$ = oxygen content of pulmonary end-capillary blood (mL/dL)

CaO_2 = oxygen content of arterial blood (mL/dL)

$C\bar{v}O_2$ = mixed venous oxygen content (mL/dL)

Venous-to-Arterial Shunt (Clinical Form)

The clinical shunt equation is a rearrangement of the classic $\dot{Q}s/\dot{Q}T$ equation, with the assumption that arterial hemoglobin is fully saturated with oxygen when the arterial oxygen tension is greater than 150 mm Hg. This assumption is valid because the test is done with an inspired oxygen fraction of 1.0, which usually results in an arterial oxygen tension greater than 150 mm Hg. In most circumstances in which this form of the equation is used, the arteriovenous content difference, $C(a-\bar{v})O_2$ is assumed to be 3.5 vol%. Figure 3–9 shows the relations between arterial blood tension and inspired oxygen concentration for different values of shunt. Table 3–6 shows "normal" values for respiratory gas exchange.

Abbreviation: $\dot{Q}s/\dot{Q}T$

Units: %

Normal value: 2–5 (children and adults)

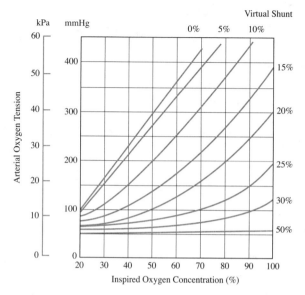

Figure 3-9 Graph relating PaO$_2$ and inspired oxygen concentration for different values of virtual shunt. Shaded lines represent hemoglobin concentration range of 10-14 g/dL and PaCO$_2$ range of 25-40 mm Hg (3.3-5.3 kPa).

Equation:

$$\frac{\dot{Q}_S}{\dot{Q}_T} = \frac{(P_{AO_2} - P_{aO_2})0.0031}{C(a-\overline{v})O_2 + (P_{AO_2} - P_{aO_2})0.0031}$$

where

$\dot{Q}_S$ = shunted portion of cardiac output

$\dot{Q}_T$ = total cardiac output

P_{AO_2} = partial pressure of oxygen in alveolar gas (mm Hg)

P_{aO_2} = partial pressure of oxygen in arterial blood (mm Hg)

0.0031 = a constant derived using the Bunsen solubility coefficient for oxygen in blood (i.e., for each 100 mL of blood at BTPS, 0.0031 mL of oxygen can be dissolved for each 1.0 mm Hg of oxygen tension)

$C(a-\overline{v})O_2$ = arteriovenous oxygen content difference (mL/dL)

Table 3-6 Respiratory Gas Exchange and Pressures

Measurement	Symbol	Adult	Infant	Units
Flows				
Alveolar ventilation	($\dot{V}_A$)	60	120	mL/kg/min
Pulmonary capillary flow	($\dot{Q}_C$)	75	200	mL/kg/min
Ventilation-perfusion ratio	($\dot{V}/\dot{Q}$)	0.8	0.6	
Venous admixture				
Shunt flow/total flow	$\dot{Q}_S/\dot{Q}_T$	0.05	0.05-0.15	
Alveolar gases				
Oxygen	($P_{A}O_2$)	105	105	mm Hg
Carbon dioxide	($P_{A}CO_2$)	40	35	mm Hg
Nitrogen	($P_{A}N_2$)	568	573	mm Hg
Arterial gases				
Oxygen	($P_{a}O_2$)	95	80	mm Hg
Carbon dioxide	($P_{a}CO_2$)	41	36	mm Hg
Nitrogen	($P_{a}N_2$)	575	583	mm Hg
Gas differences				
Oxygen	$P_{(A-a)}O_2$	10	24	mm Hg
Carbon dioxide	$P_{(A-a)}CO_2$	1	1	mm Hg
Nitrogen	$P_{(A-a)}N_2$	7	10	mm Hg

Equations for Human Blood-Oxygen Dissociation Computation

The following equations assume blood temperature = 37°C and pH = 7.40.

Oxygen Saturation (SO_2, as a Decimal Fraction) from Oxygen Tension (PO_2, in mm Hg):

$$SaO_2 = ([PO_2^3 + 150 \times PO_2)^{-1} \times 23{,}400] + 1)^{-1} \qquad (3\text{--}1)$$

PO_2 from SO_2 (for $SO_2 < 0.96$):

$$PO_2 = \exp\left[0.385 \times \ln(SO_2^{-1} - 1)^{-1} + 3.32 - (72 \times SO_2)^{-1} - \frac{(SO_2)^6}{6}\right] \qquad (3\text{--}2)$$

where

ln represents the natural logarithm (i.e., $\log_e$)

Correction of PO_2 to pH = 7.40 (Bohr Effect):

$$PO_2 \,(\text{at } 7.40) \;=\; PO_2 \times e^{1.1 \times (\text{pH} - 7.4)} \qquad (3\text{--}3)$$

Computation of P_{50}:

Step 1: Obtain a sample of blood with a measured saturation between 0.2 and 0.8.

Step 2: Measure the PO_2 and pH of the sample at 37°C.

Step 3: Use equation (3–2) above to calculate PO_2 from the measured SO_2; use this value as PO_2 (std) in equation (3–4) below.

Step 4: Use equation (3–3) above to estimate PO_2 at pH = 7.4 from the measured PO_2 and pH; use this value as PO_2 (obs) in equation (3–4) below.

Step 5: $P_{50} = \dfrac{26.7 \times PO_2(\text{obs})}{PO_2(\text{std})}$ $\qquad (3\text{--}4)$

Hemoglobin Affinity for Oxygen

(See Figure 3–10 and Figure 3–11.) Factors shifting the hemoglobin-oxygen dissociation curve to the right (decreased affinity):

1. Acidemia
2. Hyperthermia
3. Hypercarbia
4. Increased 2,3-diphosphoglycerate (2,3-DPG)

Factors shifting the hemoglobin-oxygen dissociation curve to the left (increased affinity):

1. Alkalemia
2. Hypothermia
3. Hypocarbia
4. Decreased 2,3-DPG

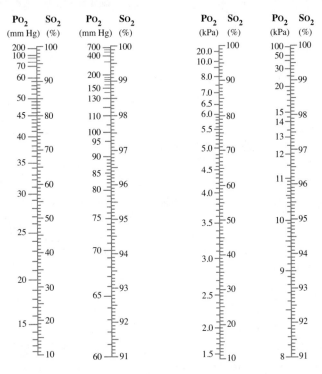

Figure 3-10 Nomogram relating Po_2 and oxygen saturation (So_2) at 37°C, pH = 7.40, and base excess = 0.

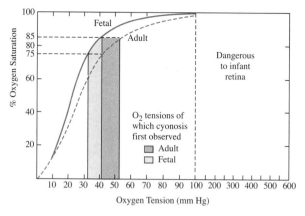

Figure 3-11 Oxyhemoglobin dissociation curves. P_{50}: An index of the affinity of hemoglobin for oxygen. It is defined as the oxygen tension at which 50% of the hemoglobin is saturated at 37°C, Pco_2 = 40 mm Hg, and pH = 7.4. The normal adult P_{50} is approximately 27 mm Hg. A reduced P_{50} means an increased hemoglobin affinity for oxygen.

■ BLOOD-GAS ANALYSIS: TRADITIONAL AND THE STEWART METHOD

Henderson-Hasselbalch Equation

This equation expresses the blood acid–base relationship in terms of the bicarbonate ion to carbonic acid ratio. It is based on the chemical equation

$$H_2CO_3 \rightarrow H^+ + HCO_3^-$$

which describes the dissociation of carbonic acid into hydrogen ions and bicarbonate ions. The law of mass action defines the dissociation constant (K_a) of carbonic acid as

$$K_a = \frac{[H^+][HCO_3^-]}{[H_2CO_3]}$$

The carbonic acid concentration is dependent on the amount of dissolved carbon dioxide in the blood. The amount of dissolved carbon dioxide (mmol/L) is dependent on its solubility coefficient (0.03 mmol/L/mm Hg) and the partial pressure of carbon dioxide in the blood (Pco_2) (see Figure 3–16). Thus, the above equation can be written as

$$K_a = \frac{[H^+][HCO_3^-]}{0.03 P_{CO_2}}$$

This equation can now be rearranged to a more useful form that relates plasma hydrogen ion concentration, P_{CO_2}, and bicarbonate concentration, all measurable quantities:

$$[H^+] = K_a\left(\frac{0.03 P_{CO_2}}{[HCO_3^-]}\right)$$

The hydrogen ion concentration is more commonly expressed in terms of pH (negative log of hydrogen ion concentration) as follows:

$$-\log[H^+] = -\log K_a - \log\left(\frac{0.03 P_{CO_2}}{[HCO_3^-]}\right)$$

$$pH = -\log K_a + \log\left(\frac{[HCO_3^-]}{0.03 P_{CO_2}}\right)$$

The value of $-\log K_a$ (i.e., PK_a) is 6.1. Substituting normal values for HCO_3^- (24 mmol/L) and $P_{A CO_2}$ (40 mm Hg) in the above equation yields

$$pH = 6.1 + \log\left(\frac{24}{0.03 \times 40}\right)$$

$$= 6.1 + 1.3$$

$$\therefore \text{ normal pH } = 7.4.$$

Table 3–7 shows the ranges for pH and $P_{A CO_2}$ at sea level. Table 3–8 shows the formulas used to calculate the expected compensation in simple acid–base disorders. Figures 3–12, 3–13, 3–14, and 3–15 depict nomograms, flow charts, and maps to interpret acid–base disorders.

Table 3-7 Ranges and Nomenclature for pH and $P_{A CO_2}$

	pH	$P_{A CO_2}$ (mm Hg)
Normal range		
Mean	7.40	40
1 SD	7.38-7.42	38-42
2 SD	7.35-7.45	35-45
Alkalemia	≥7.46	
Acidemia	≤7.34	

Table 3-8 Expected Compensation for Simple Acid-Base Disorders

Disorder and Compensation	pH	Initial Change	Compensatory Change	Anion Gap
Metabolic acidosis	↓	↓ HCO_3^-	↓ $Paco_2$	N, ↑
$Paco_2 = (1.5 \times HCO) + 8 \pm 2$				
$Paco_2 \approx$ last two digits of pH				
$Paco_2 \downarrow$ 1.0-1.5 torr/ $\downarrow$ 1.0 mEq/L HCO_3^-				
Metabolic alkalosis	↑	↑ HCO_3^-	↑ $Paco_2$	N, ↓
$Paco_2 = (0.7 \times HCO_3^-) + 21$				
$Paco_2 = 40 + (0.6 \times$ standard base excess)				
$Paco_2 \uparrow$ 0.5-1.0 torr/ $\uparrow$ 1 mEq/L HCO_3^-				
Respiratory acidosis	↓	↑ $Paco_2$	↑ HCO_3^-	N
Acute (<24 h)				
$\Delta H^+ = 0.8 \times \Delta Paco_2$				
$\Delta pH = 0.008 \times \Delta Paco_2$				
$HCO_3^- = ([Paco_2 - 40]/10) + 24$				
$HCO_3^- \uparrow$ 0.1-1.0 mEq/L/ $\uparrow$ 10 torr $Paco_2$				
Chronic (>24 h)				
$\Delta H^+ = 0.3 \times \Delta Paco_2$				
$\Delta pH = 0.003 \times \Delta Paco_2$				
$HCO_3^- = ([Paco_2 - 40]/3) + 24$				
$HCO_3^- \uparrow$ 1.1-3.5 mEq/L/ $\uparrow$ 10 torr $Paco_2$				
Respiratory alkalosis	↑	↓ $Paco_2$	↓ HCO_3^-	N, ↑
Acute (<12 h)				
$\Delta H^+ = 0.8 \times \Delta Paco_2$				
$HCO_3^- = 24 - ([40 - Paco_2]/5)$				
$HCO_3^- \downarrow$ 0-2.0 mEq/L/ $\downarrow$ 10 torr $Paco_2$				
Chronic (12-72 h)				
$\Delta H^+ = 0.17 \times \Delta Paco_2$				
$HCO_3^- = 24 - ([40 - Paco_2]/2)$				
$HCO_3^- \downarrow$ 2.1-5.0 mEq/L/ $\downarrow$ 10 torr $Paco_2$				

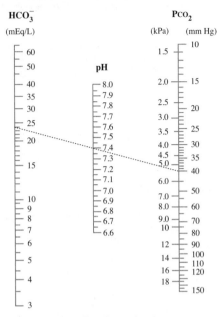

Figure 3-12 Modified Siggaard-Anderson nomogram relating blood pH, bicarbonate concentration (HCO_3^-), and Pco_2.

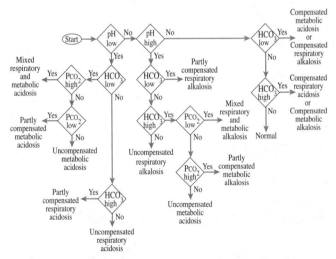

Figure 3-13 Flow chart illustrating a simplified acid-base interpretation scheme.

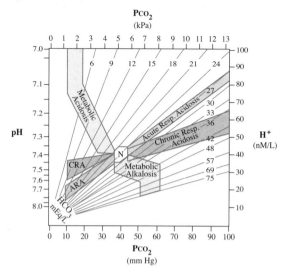

Figure 3-14 An acid-base map for children and adults. N = normal acid-base status; CRA = chronic respiratory alkalosis; ARA = acute respiratory alkalosis.

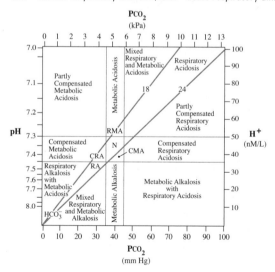

Figure 3-15 An acid-base map for neonates. RMA = mixed respiratory and metabolic acidosis; N = normal acid-base status; CRA = compensated respiratory alkalosis; CMA = compensated metabolic alkalosis; RA = respiratory alkalosis.

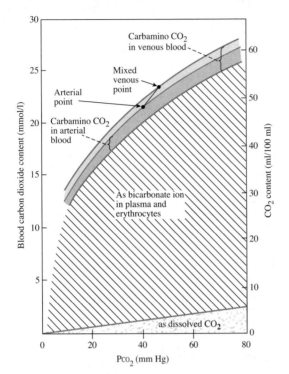

Figure 3-16 Components of carbon dioxide curve for whole blood.

Anion Gap

The anion gap is used to evaluate the nature of a metabolic acidosis. In disease states characterized by elevated organic acids, the anion gap increases. The anion gap decreases 2.3 to 2.5 mEq/L for every 1 g/dL albumin reduction in plasma.

Abbreviation: AG

Units: mEq/L

Normal value: 15–20

Equations:

$$AG = (Na^+ + K^+) - (Cl^- + HCO_3^-)$$

or

$$AG = Na^+ - (Cl^- + HCO_3^-) \qquad \text{(normal range 8–12)}$$

or

$$adjAG = [(Na^+ + K^+) - (Cl^- + HCO_3^-) + (2.5 \times ([\text{normal albumin}] - [\text{observed albumin}]))$$

or

$$AGc = ([Na^+ + K^+] - [Cl^- + HCO_3^-]) - ([2 \times \text{albumin}] + [0.5 \times \text{phosphate}]) - \text{lactate} \qquad \text{(normal range is 0)}$$

where

adjAG = albumin-adjusted anion gap

AGc = anion gap corrected

Na^+ = serum sodium concentration (mEq/L)

K^+ = serum potassium concentration (mEq/L)

Cl^- = serum chloride concentration (mEq/L)

HCO_3^- = serum bicarbonate concentration (mEq/L)

Albumin (g/dL)

Phosphate (mg/dL)

Lactate (md/dL)

Delta-Delta Gap

A ratio used to evaluate mixed acid–base disorders. It is based on the buffer concept that for every molecule of acid added to the extracellular fluid, the acid will react with HCO_3^- to produce water and CO_2. Hence, one expects that for every acid molecule produced, one bicarbonate molecule should decrease. *Note:* The ratio depends on how the acid is buffered. Lactic acid ratio is 1.6/1, and ketones 1:1.

Abbreviation: Δ/Δ

Units: mEq/L

Normal value: 1–2

Equation:

$$\Delta/\Delta = \frac{AG_{measured} - AG_{normal}}{HCO_3^-{}_{normal} - HCO_3^-{}_{measured}}$$

where

AG = anion gap (mEq/L)

HCO_3^- = serum bicarbonate concentration (mEq/L)

Base Excess

The amount of acid or base that must be added to a sample of whole blood *in vitro* to restore the pH to 7.40 while the P_{ACO_2} is held at 40 mmHg. It represents the quantity of metabolic acidosis or alkalosis. To enhance the behavior of the formula *in vivo*, the standard base excess (SBE) standardizes the effect of hemoglobin on CO_2 titration. Further corrections (corrected SBE) take into account albumin and phosphate yielding the closest behavior to actual physiology.

Abbreviation: BE, SBE, and SBEc

Units: mEq/L

Normal value: ±2

Equations:

$$BE = (HCO_3^- - 24.4 + [2.3 \times Hb + 7.7] \times [pH - 7.4]) \times (1 - 0.023 \times Hb)$$

or

$$SBE = 0.9287 \times (HCO_3^- - 24.4 + [2.3 \times Hb + 14.83 \times [pH - 7.4]])$$

or

$$SBEc = (HCO_3^- - 24.4) + ([8.3 \times albumin \times 0.15] + [0.29 \times phosphate \times 0.32]) \times (pH - 7.4)$$

where

BE = base excess (mEq/L)

SBE = standard base excess (mEq/L)

HCO_3^- = serum bicarbonate concentration (mEq/L)

Hb = hemoglobin (mmol/L) (1 mmol/L = 0.1 mg/dL Hb)

pH = power of hydrogen (dimensionless)

Albumin (g/dL)

Phosphate (mg/dL)

Stewart Approach to Acid–Base Disorders

Peter A. Stewart introduced in 1981 an alternative view to the interpretation of acid–base theory. His view expressed that acid–base physiology has independent and dependent variables. The dependent variables ($[H^+]$, $[OH^-]$, $[HCO_3^-]$, $[CO_3^{-2}]$, $[HA]$, $[A^-]$) are controlled by the independent variables (P_{CO_2}, total weak nonvolatile acids and the strong ion difference). Thus, departing from the concept that HCO_3^- and pH are controlled directly, and establishing the mathematical bases to explain the control by the independent variables.

There are six equations that describe the interactions between dependent and independent variables:

1. Water dissociation equilibrium

$$[H^+] \times [OH^-] = K'_w$$

2. Weak acid dissociation equilibrium

$$[H^+] \times [A^-] = K_a x\, [HA]$$

3. Conservation of mass for A

$$[A_{TOT}] = [HA] + [A^-]$$

4. Bicarbonate ion formation equilibrium

$$[H^+] \times [HCO_3^-] = K'_1 \times S \times P_{CO_2}$$

5. Carbonate ion formation equilibrium

$$[H^+] \times [CO_3^{-2}] = K_3 \times [HCO_3^-]$$

6. Electrical charge equation

$$[SID^+] = [HCO_3^-] + [A^-] + [CO_3^{-2}] + [OH^-] - [H^+]$$

where

$[A^-]$ = dissociated weak acid concentration, mostly albumin and phosphate

$[HA]$ = concentration of weak acid associated with a proton

K'_w = autoionization constant for water

K_a = weak acid dissociation constant for HA

$[A_{TOT}]$ = total concentration of weak nonvolatile acids, inorganic phosphate, serum proteins, and albumin

K'_1 = apparent equilibrium constant for the Henderson–Hasselbach equation

S = solubility of CO_2 in plasma

K_3 = apparent equilibrium dissociation constant for bicarbonate

SID^+ = strong ion difference (see below)

Strong Ion Difference (SID)

The difference in strong ions ($[Na^+ + K^+] - [Cl^- + lactate]$). In practice, this is incalculable because we are unable to measure all strong ions. However, calculations to obtain the apparent and the effective difference are available. The apparent SID is directly calculated from available strong cations and anions in blood. The effective SID (conceptually the same as the known buffer base) is calculated with the CO_2, albumin, and phosphate.

Abbreviation: $[SID^+]_a$ and $[SID^+]_e$

Units: mEq/L

Normal value: SID = 40 mEq

Equations:

$$[SID^+]_a = [Na^+] + [K^+] + [Mg^{++}] + [Ca^{++}] - [Cl^-]$$
$$- [lactate] - [other strong anions]$$
$$[SID^+]_e = [HCO_3^-] + [A^-]$$

where

Mg^+ = ionized magnesium concentration (mEq/L)

Ca^{++} = ionized calcium (mEq/L)

$[A^-]$ = concentration of dissociated weak noncarbonic acids, principally albumin and phosphate

Strong Ion Gap (SIG)

The difference between the effective and apparent SID. The SIG may better represent the amount of unmeasured anions, when compared to the anion gap. A particular example is when the albumin is low, the SIG may be high (a manifestation of unmeasured anions) while the anion gap is normal.

> Abbreviation: SIG
>
> Units: mEq/L
>
> Normal value: 0

Equation:

$$SIG = [SID^+]_a - [SID^+]_e$$

Based on these concepts, acid–base disorders can be classified using the independent variables ($Paco_2$ and A_{TOT} and SID). See Table 3–9.

Table 3-9 Classification of Acid-Base Disorders Based on Stewart Independent Variables

Respiratory
Changes in $Paco_2$ produce expected changes in [H^+]
Metabolic
1. Change in [SID]
a. Change in concentration
i. Dehydration: Concentrates alkalinity and increases [SID]
ii. H_2O overload: Dilutes alkalinity and decreases [SID]
b. Changes in strong ion concentrations
i. Inorganic acids: Increase in chloride (low [SID] and low SIG)
ii. Organic acids: Accumulation of lactate, formate, or ketones (low [SID] and high SIG)
2. Change in [A_{TOT}]
Changes in concentration of phosphate, albumin, and other plasma proteins.

Data from Corey, H. E. et al. *Critical Care* 9 (2005), 184-192.

■ HEMODYNAMICS

Cardiac Output

Cardiac output equals heart rate times stroke volume. Thus, cardiac output may be increased by increasing either heart rate or stroke volume. Increasing the heart rate is the most rapid method of increasing cardiac output, which can double or triple in a healthy person.

Abbreviation: CO

Unit: L/min

Normal value: 4.0–8.0 (adults); cardiac output for all patients can be found by multiplying normal cardiac index by body surface area (BSA).

Cardiac Output (Fick Principle)

This equation is valid if two blood samples (arterial and mixed venous blood) are drawn simultaneously during mixed expired gas collection and assume a steady state of ventilation and circulation.

Abbreviation: $\dot{Q}$

Units: L/min

Normal value: 4.0–8.0 (adult)

Equation:

$$\dot{Q} = \frac{\dot{V}O_2}{(CaO_2 - C\overline{V}O_2) \times 10}$$

where

$\dot{V}O_2$ = (mL/min STPD)

CaO_2 = arterial oxygen content (mL/dL)

$C\overline{V}O_2$ = mixed venous oxygen content (mL/dL)

Cardiac Index

Cardiac output varies with body size and has been shown to increase in proportion to the surface area of the body. The cardiac index (cardiac output per square meter of BSA) is therefore useful in comparing the cardiac outputs of different-sized people. All flow-related hemodynamic variables can be indexed by substituting cardiac index for cardiac output in their equations.

Abbreviation: CI

Units: L/min/m^2

Normal value: 2.7–4.5 (children and adults)

Equation:

$$CI = CO/BSA$$

where

CO = cardiac output (L/min)

BSA = body surface area (m^2)

Stroke Volume

The volume that the left ventricle ejects with each contraction. It is influenced by (1) cardiac contractility, (2) ventricular end-diastolic volume (preload), and (3) impedance to left ventricular outflow (afterload).

Abbreviation: SV

Units: mL/beat

Normal value: 60–130 (adults)

Equation:

$$SV = \frac{CO \times 1000}{HR}$$

where

CO = cardiac output (L/min)

HR = heart rate (bpm)

Stroke Index

Abbreviation: SI

Units: mL/beat/m^2

Normal value: 30–50 (children and adults)

Equation:

$$SI = \frac{CI \times 1000}{HR}$$

where

CI = cardiac index (L/min/m^2)

HR = heart rate (bpm)

Mean Arterial Pressure

The average blood pressure. It represents the force that drives the blood through the systemic circulatory system. Thus, it is this parameter that is important from the perspective of tissue blood flow. The mean arterial pressure is directly proportional to the cardiac output and the systemic vascular resistance. Any change in cardiac output (provided the resistance stays constant), either by stroke volume or heart rate, will cause a corresponding change in mean arterial pressure.

Abbreviation: MAP

Units: mm Hg

Normal value: 82–102 (adults)

Equations:

$$MAP \cong 1/3(\text{systolic} - \text{diastolic}) + \text{diastolic}$$

or

$$MAP \cong \frac{(\text{systolic} + 2 \times \text{diastolic})}{3}$$

or

$$MAP = (CO \times SVR) + CVP$$

where

CO = cardiac output (L/min)

SVR = systemic vascular resistance

CVP = central venous pressure

Central Venous Pressure

Abbreviation: CVP

Units: mm Hg

Normal value: 1–7 (adults)

Table 3-10 Hemodynamic Parameters

Intracardiac Pressure Values Location		Pressure* (mm Hg)
Right atrium		
	Mean	−2-6
Right ventricle		
	Systolic	14-38
	Diastolic	0-7
Pulmonary artery		
	Systolic	12-28
	Diastolic	4-12
	Mean	6-18
Pulmonary artery occlusion pressure		
	Mean	6-12
Left atrium		
	Mean	6-12
Left ventricle		
	Systolic	81-141
	Diastolic	3-11

*Based on normal patients aged 2 months to 20 years.

Vascular Resistance

The opposition to blood flow in a vessel. Vascular resistance cannot be measured directly but is calculated from measurements of blood flow and pressure. Resistance is defined as

$$R = \Delta P / \dot{Q}$$

where

R = resistance

ΔP = the difference in pressure between two points in a vessel

$\dot{Q}$ = the flow of blood through a vessel

When $\Delta P = 1$ mm Hg and flow is 1 mL/sec, then R is said to be 1 resistance unit. Resistance may also be expressed as a basic physical unit in the centimeter-gram-second (CGS) system of measurement. The units of resistance in this system are dyne $\cdot$ s/cm^5 and may be calculated from pressure and flow measurements by the following formula:

$$\text{dyne} \cdot \text{s/cm}^5 = \frac{(1333)(\text{mm Hg})}{\text{mL/s}} = \frac{(79.92)(\text{mm Hg})}{\text{L/min}}$$

where

1333 = the factor to convert mm Hg to dyne/cm^2

To convert from "units" to dyne $\cdot$ s/cm^5, simply multiply the number of units by 79.92 (80 is not used in most texts).

Systemic Vascular Resistance

Abbreviation: SVR

Normal value: 900–1600 dyne $\cdot$ s/cm^5 (adults)

Equation:

$$\text{SVR (units)} = \frac{\text{MAP} - \text{CVP}}{\text{CO}}$$

where

MAP = mean arterial pressure (mm Hg)
CVP = central venous (or mean right atrial) pressure (mm Hg)
CO = cardiac output (L/min)

Systemic Vascular Resistance Index

Abbreviation: SVRI

Normal value: 1760–2600 dyne $\cdot$ s/cm^5/m^2 (children and adults)
10–15 units/m^2 (infants)
15–30 units/m^2 (children and adolescents)

Equation:

$$\text{SVRI (units)} = \frac{\text{MPA} - \text{CVP}}{\text{CI}}$$

where

MAP = mean arterial pressure (mm Hg)
CVP = central venous (or mean right atrial) pressure (mm Hg)
CI = cardiac index (L/min/m^2)

Pulmonary Vascular Resistance

Abbreviation: PVR

Normal value: <160 dyne $\cdot$ s/cm^5, <2 units (adults)

Equation:

$$PVR \text{ (units)} = \frac{MPAP - PAOP}{CO}$$

where

MPAP = mean pulmonary artery pressure (mm Hg)
PAOP = pulmonary artery occlusion pressure or mean left atrial pressure
        (mm Hg)
CO = cardiac output (L/min)

Pulmonary Vascular Resistance Index

Abbreviation: PVRI

Normal value: 45–225 dyne $\cdot$ s/cm^5/m^2 (children and adults)
                8–10 unit/m^2 (newborn)
                3 unit/m^2 (infants)

Equation:

$$PVR \text{ (units)} = \frac{MPAP - PAOP}{CI}$$

where

MPAP = mean pulmonary artery pressure (mm Hg)
PAOP = pulmonary artery occlussion pressure or mean left atrial
        pressure (mm Hg)
CI = cardiac index (L/min/m^2)

Coronary Perfusion Pressure

For mean aortic diastolic pressures between 40 and 80 mm Hg, coronary circulation is nearly a linear function of perfusion pressure at the coronary ostia. Coronary artery collapse occurs at approximately 40 mm Hg. Therefore, coronary artery perfusion pressure should be maintained at 60 to 80 mm Hg.

Equation:

Coronary perfusion pressure = arterial diastolic pressure − LVEDP

where

LVEDP = left ventricular end-diastolic pressure (mm Hg) and

LVEDP $\approx$ pulmonary artery occlusion pressure

Cerebral Perfusion Pressure

Abbreviation: CPP

Units: mm Hg

Normal value: 70–110

Equation:

$$CPP = MAP - ICP$$

where

MAP = mean arterial pressure (mm Hg)

ICP = intracranial pressure (mm Hg)

Stroke Work

The product of the amount of blood ejected from a ventricle multiplied by the average pressure generated during that heartbeat. It is a parameter used in evaluating the pumping function of the heart.

Left Ventricular Stroke Work Index

Abbreviation: LVSWI

Units: $g \cdot m/m^2$

Normal value: 42–64 (children and adults)

Equation:

$$\text{LVSWI} = \text{SI} \times (\text{MAP} - \text{PAOP}) \times 0.0136 \approx \text{SI} \times \text{MAP} \times 0.0136$$

where

SI = stroke index (mL/m^2)

MAP = mean arterial pressure (mm Hg)

PAOP = pulmonary artery occlusion pressure (mm Hg)

Left Cardiac Work Index

Abbreviation: LCWI

Units: kg · m/m^2/min

Normal value: 2.8–4.3 (children and adults)

Equation:

$$\text{LCWI} = \text{CI} \times (\text{MAP} - \text{PAOP}) \times 0.0136 \approx \text{CI} \times \text{MAP} \times 0.0136$$

where

CI = cardiac index (L/min/m^2)

MAP = mean arterial pressure (mm Hg)

PAOP = pulmonary artery occlusion pressure (mm Hg)

Right Ventricular Stroke Work Index

Abbreviation: RVSWI

Units: g · m/m^2

Normal units: 3.8–7.6 (children and adults)

Equation:

$$\text{RVSWI} = \text{SI} \times (\text{MPAP} - \text{CVP}) \times 0.0136 \approx \text{SI} \times \text{MPAP} \times 0.0136$$

where

SI = stroke index (mL/m^2)

MPAP = mean pulmonary artery pressure (mm Hg)

CVP = central venous pressure (mm Hg)

Right Cardiac Work Index

Abbreviation: RCWI
Unit: $kg \cdot m/m^2/min$
Normal value: 0.4–0.6 (children and adults)

Equation:

$$RCWI = CI \times (MPAP - CVP) \times 0.0136 \approx CI \times MPAP \times 0.0136,$$

where

CI = cardiac index $(L/min/m^2)$
MPAP = mean pulmonary artery pressure (mm Hg)
CVP = central venous pressure (mm Hg)

Oxygen Availability (Delivery)

Oxygen availability (sometimes called oxygen delivery) is the total amount of oxygen potentially available for tissue consumption per unit time.

Abbreviation: O_2AV, DO_2, $\dot{Q}O_2$
 DO_2I (indexed to BSA)
Unit: $mL/min/m^2$ (STPD) for DO_2I, mL/min for DO_2
Normal value: $DO_2 = $ 950–1150 mL/min
 $DO_2I = $ 520–720 $mL/min/m^2$

Equations:

$$DO_2 = CaO_2 \times CO \times 10$$
$$DO_2I = CaO_2 \times CI \times 10$$

where

CaO_2 = arterial oxygen content (mL/dL)
CI = cardiac index $(L/min/m^2)$
CO = cardiac output (L/min)

Note: Brain hypoxia is probable when O_2AV drops below 450 $mL/min/m^2$.

Oxygen Consumption

The amount of oxygen extracted from the blood by the tissues. Oxygen consumption may be limited by the oxygen availability or by tissue extraction (e.g., as in cyanide poisoning). See Tables 3–11 and 3–12.

Abbreviation: $\dot{V}O_2$ and $\dot{V}O_2I$ (indexed to BSA)
Units: $mL/min/m^2$ (STPD) for $\dot{V}O_2I$, mL/min for $\dot{V}O_2$
Normal value: $\dot{V}O_2I = $ 100–180 (children and adults)
 $\dot{V}O_2 = $ 200–250

Table 3-11 Oxygen Consumption (mL/min/m²) as a Function of Age and Heart Rate for Males

Age (yr)	Heart Rate (bpm)										
	50	60	70	80	90	100	110	120	130	140	150
3				156	159	163	167	171	175	178	182
4			149	152	156	160	164	168	171	175	179
6		140	144	148	152	155	159	163	167	170	174
8		137	141	144	148	152	156	160	163	167	171
10	131	134	138	142	146	149	153	157	161	165	168
12	128	132	136	140	144	147	151	155	159	162	166
14	127	130	134	138	142	14	149	153	157	161	164
16	125	129	133	136	140	144	148	152	155	159	163
18	124	128	131	135	139	143	146	150	154	158	162
20	123	126	130	134	138	141	145	149	153	157	160
25	120	124	128	131	135	139	143	146	150	154	158
30	118	122	125	129	133	137	141	144	148	152	156
35	116	120	124	127	131	135	139	143	146	150	
40	115	118	122	126	130	134	137	141	145	149	

Equations:

$$\dot{V}O_2 = (CaO_2 - C\overline{v}O_2) \times CO_4 \times 10$$

$$\dot{V}O_2 = (CaO_2 - C\overline{v}O_2) \times CI \times 10$$

where

CaO_2 = arterial oxygen content (mL/dL)

$C\overline{v}O_2$ = mixed venous oxygen content (mL/dL)

Prediction Equations:
Males:

$$\dot{V}O_2 = 138.1 - 11.49 \times \ln (age) + 0.378 \times (heart\ rate)$$

Females:

$$\dot{V}O_2 = 138.1 - 17.04 \times \ln (age) + 0.378 \times (heart\ rate)$$

Table 3-12 Oxygen Consumption (mL/min/m^2) as a Function of Age and Heart Rate for Females

Age (yr)	Heart Rate (bpm)										
	50	60	70	80	90	100	110	120	130	140	150
				150	153	157	161	165	169	172	176
			141	145	148	152	156	160	164	167	171
		130	134	138	142	145	149	153	157	160	164
		125	129	133	137	140	144	148	152	156	159
10	118	122	125	129	133	137	140	144	148	152	156
12	115	118	122	126	130	134	137	141	145	149	152
14	112	116	120	123	127	131	135	138	142	146	150
16	110	114	117	121	125	129	132	136	140	144	148
18	108	112	115	119	123	127	130	134	138	142	146
20	106	110	114	117	121	125	129	132	136	140	144
25	102	106	110	113	117	121	125	129	132	136	140
30	99	103	107	110	114	118	122	126	129	133	137
35	96	100	104	108	112	115	119	123	127	130	
40	94	98	102	105	109	113	117	121	124	128	

where

heart rate is in beats per minute

ln represents the natural logarithm (i.e., log$_e$)

Oxygen Extraction Ratio

A ratio of the oxygen consumption to the oxygen availability and an indicator of the body's metabolic level (for a given cardiac output). Conversely, given a stable level of hemoglobin, arterial saturation, and oxygen consumption, an increasing oxygen extraction ratio indicated a fall in cardiac output.

Abbreviation: O$_2$ER

Units: %

Normal value: 22–30 (children and adults)

Equation:

$$O_2ER = \frac{(CaO_2 - C\overline{v}O_2)}{CaO_2}$$

where

CaO_2 = arterial oxygen content (mL/dL)

$C\overline{v}O_2$ = mixed venous oxygen content (mL/dL)

Oxygen Extraction Index

Abbreviation: O_2EI

Units: %

Normal value: 22–25%

Equation:

$$O_2EI = \frac{(SaO_2 - S\overline{v}O_2)}{SaO_2}$$

where

SaO_2 = Oxygen saturation of arteral blood

$S\overline{v}O_2$ = Oxygen saturation of mixed venous blood

4

Gas Therapy

For the respiratory care practitioner to provide gas therapy effectively, it is necessary to understand the physics of gases. This chapter will describe the relationships among pressure, temperature, mass, and volume for most medical gases. This chapter will also describe the packaging, distribution, and conversion equations that permit the practitioner to use these gases effectively.

■ THE GENERAL GAS LAW

The behavior of an ideal gas is governed by the interdependent relationships of four thermodynamic variables: mass, pressure, volume, and absolute temperature. The equation relating these variables is called the ideal gas law and is written as

$$PV = nRT$$

where

P = absolute pressure of dry gas in atmospheres (atm)

V = volume in liters (L)

n = moles of gas

R = the universal gas constant: $(0.0821 \text{ L} \cdot \text{atm/mole} \cdot \text{K})$

T = absolute temperature in degrees Kelvin (K)

Since water vapor in a saturated mixture does not act like an ideal gas, the preceding equation is applied to the dry gas portion of the mixture. If a gas is saturated with water vapor, at a given temperature its dry gas pressure is obtained by subtracting the water vapor at that temperature.

In situations where mass (i.e., number of moles) remains constant, the general gas law is often simplified to $PV/T = k$, where k is a constant. Furthermore, the general gas law is most often utilized to correct for the volume change when pressure and temperature are changed. We would use the *combined gas law* form:

$$\frac{P_1V_1}{T_1} = \frac{P_2V_2}{T_2}$$

A common and useful application of the combined general gas law is converting gas volumes from room temperature (ATPS) to body conditions (BTPS).

Problem:

Correct a measured vital capacity of 4.8 L to BTPS given that the patient's body temperature is normal and the pulmonary function laboratory is at sea level with a room temperature of 25°C.

Solution:

Condition 1 = ATPS

$$P_1 = P_B - P_{H_2O}$$
$$= 760 - 23.8 \text{ (at } 25°C)$$
$$= 736.2 \text{ mm Hg}$$
$$V_1 = 4.8 \text{ L}$$
$$T_1 = 25°C + 273 = 298 \text{ K}$$

Condition 2 = BTPS

$$P_2 = 760 - 47 \text{ (at } 37°C)$$
$$= 713 \text{ mm Hg}$$
$$V_2 = \text{unknown value}$$
$$T_2 = 37°C + 273 = 310 \text{ K}$$

We derive the formula for converting gas volume from ATPS to BTPS by solving the combined gas law for V_2,

$$\frac{P_1 V_1}{T_1} = \frac{P_2 V_2}{T_2}$$

$$V_2 = \frac{P_1 V_1 T_2}{T_1 P_2}$$

and substituting the known values:

$$V_2 = \frac{732.2 \times 4.8 \times 310}{298 \times 713}$$

$$= 5.2 \text{ L}$$

■ SPECIAL GAS LAWS

Boyle's Law

If temperature and mass remain constant, the volume of a gas varies inversely with the pressure applied to that gas. Symbolically,

$$V = \frac{k}{P}$$

or, equivalently,

$$P_1V_1 = P_2V_2$$

where

k is a constant

Problem:

Consider a syringe filled with a certain amount of dry gas. If the outlet is blocked while the plunger is depressed, the pressure of the gas inside the syringe will rise as its volume decreases (we assume that there are no leaks and that the temperature change of the gas is negligible). If the gauge pressure of the gas is 30 cm H_2O when the volume of the gas is 40 mL, what will the pressure be when the gas is compressed to 35 mL?

Solution:

Condition 1:

P_1 (absolute) = gauge pressure + atmospheric pressure

30 cm H_2O = 22 mm Hg

P_1 = 22 + 760 = 782 mm Hg

V_1 = 40 mL

Condition 2:

P_2 = unknown value

V_2 = 35 mL

Solving Boyle's law for the unknown variable gives

$$P_1V_1 = P_2V_2$$

$$P_2 = \frac{P_1V_1}{V_2}$$

$$= 782 \times \frac{40}{35}$$

$$= 894 \text{ mm Hg}$$

$$P_2 \text{ (gauge)} = (894 - 760) \times 1.36$$

$$= 182 \text{ cm } H_2O$$

Another example of Boyle's law is the effect of altitude changes on the volume of trapped gas (e.g., a pneumothorax), as shown in Table 4–1.

Table 4-1 The Effect of Altitude on Trapped Gas

Altitude		
(ft)	(m)	Expansion
10,000	3,048	150%
18,000	5,486	200%
27,000	8,230	300%
33,000	10,058	400%
38,500	11,735	500%

Charles's Law

If pressure and mass remain constant, the volume of a gas varies directly with the temperature of that gas. The equations are

$$V = kT$$

or, equivalently,

$$\frac{V_1}{T_1} = \frac{V_2}{T_2}$$

where

k is a constant

Problem:

Suppose a certain quantity of helium occupies a volume of 6.0 L at a room temperature of 22°C. If the same mass of helium were heated to 37°C, what would its new volume be?

Solution:

Condition 1:

$V_1 = 6.0$ L

$T_1 = 22°C + 273 = 295$ K

Condition 2:

$V_2 = $ unknown value

$T_2 = 37°C + 273 = 310$ K

Solving the above equation for the unknown quantity, we obtain

$$\frac{V_1}{T_1} = \frac{V_2}{T_2}$$

$$V_2 = \frac{V_1 T_2}{T_1}$$

Substituting the known quantities gives

$$V_2 = 6.0 \times \frac{310}{295}$$

$$= 6.3 \text{ L}$$

Gay-Lussac's Law

If volume and mass remain constant, the pressure of a gas varies directly with the temperature of that gas. Thus,

$$P = k\text{T}$$

or

$$\frac{P_1}{T_1} = \frac{P_2}{T_2}$$

where

k is a constant

Problem:

A common example occurs at those institutions in the northern latitude that store their gas cylinders outside. If an H cylinder of oxygen was filled to 2200 psi at room temperature (22°C), what is its pressure at −10°C?

Solution:

Condition 1:

$$P_1 \text{ (absolute)} = \text{gauge pressure} + \text{atmospheric pressure}$$
$$P_1 = 2200 \text{ psi} + 14.7 \approx 2215 \text{ psi}$$
$$T_1 = 22°C + 273 = 295 \text{ K}$$

Condition 2:

$$P_2 = \text{unknown value}$$
$$T_1 = -10°C + 273 = 263 \text{ K}$$

Using the preceding equation, we solve for the unknown pressure:

$$\frac{P_1}{T_1} = \frac{P_2}{T_2}$$

$$P_2 = \frac{P_1 T_2}{T_1}$$

Substituting the known values gives

$$P_2 = 2215 \times 263/295$$

$$= 1975 \text{ psi}$$

$$P_2 \text{ (gauge)} = 1975 - 15$$

$$= 1960 \text{ psi/gauge pressure}$$

Avogadro's Law

If pressure and temperature remain constant, the mass of a gas varies directly with the volume of that gas:

$$n = kV$$

or, equivalently,

$$\frac{n_1}{V_1} = \frac{n_2}{V_2}$$

where

k is a constant

n is the number of moles of the gas

From these equations it follows that equal volumes of gases at the same pressure and temperature have the same number of moles. Furthermore, one gram molecular weight of a gas (i.e., the atomic weight of the molecule expressed in grams) occupies 22.4 L at STPD and contains 6.02×10^{23} molecules. Avogadro's law provides the basis for the derivation of the density (mass per unit volume) of a gas. For example, the density of oxygen (ρO_2) is its gram molecular weight (gmw) divided by 22.4 L:

$$1 \text{ gmw } O_2 = 16 \times 2 \times 1 \text{ g} = 32 \text{ g}$$

$$\rho O_2 = 32/22.4 = 1.43 \text{ g/L at STPD.}$$

Specific gravity is a ratio of densities. Usually, gas densities are compared to air ($\rho_{AIR} = 1.28$ g/L at STPD). Calculation of specific gravity for oxygen reveals that it is heavier than air:

$$\text{specific gravity of } O_2 = \frac{1.43 \text{ g/L}}{1.28 \text{ g/L}}$$

$$\text{or} = 1.12$$

It is this property of oxygen that causes the "layering" of oxygen in tents, making the F_{IO_2} at the bottom of the canopy higher than at the top.

Dalton's Law of Partial Pressures

The total pressure of a gas mixture is equal to the sum of the partial pressures of the constituent gases. The partial pressure of each gas is the pressure it would exert if it occupied the entire volume alone:

$$P_{Total} = P_1 + P_2 + P_3 + \cdots + P_n$$

The partial pressure of each gas is proportional to its molar concentration in the mixture:

$$P_g = F_g \times P_{Total}$$

where

$\quad$ P_g is the partial pressure of the gas

$\quad$ F_g is the fractional concentration of the gas in the mixture

Dalton's law is important because it allows us to calculate the partial pressures of various inhaled gases. The physiologic effects of each component of inhaled air depend on the partial pressure of the component in the lungs rather than on the total pressure.

As a rough approximation, the partial pressure (in kPa) is close to the concentration (in %) at normal barometric pressure. Partial pressure in mm Hg can be approximated by multiplying the concentration (in %) by 7. For example, the P_{O_2} of air is approximately $21 \times 7 = 147$ mm Hg.

Poiseuille's Law

Poiseuille's law describes the mechanics of laminar fluid flow through a tube.

$$\dot{V} = \frac{P\pi r^4}{8\eta l}$$

where

$\dot{V}$ = flow in cm^3/s

P = pressure difference across the ends of the tube (dyne/cm^2)

π = 3.1416 . . .

r = radius of tube (cm)

l = length of tube (cm)

η = viscosity in poise (dyne · s/cm^2)

The preceding equation indicates that the pressure difference is directly proportional to the gas flow rate. Thus, for any flow rate, the pressure difference divided by the flow rate equals a constant. This constant is called resistance (R) and is defined as

$$R = \frac{8\eta l}{\pi r^4} = \frac{P}{\dot{V}}$$

The clinical significance of this definition centers around the importance of tube radius. For instance, if the radius of an airway is halved, the airway resistance in that section increases 16-fold. Bronchospasm and mucous obstruction are two frequently encountered clinical conditions that reduce airway caliber (increasing airway resistance), resulting in a rise in proximal airway pressure during volume control ventilation or acute hypoventilation during pressure control ventilation.

Another important point about this definition is that the only property of the gas that influences resistance during laminar flow is viscosity. This is in contrast to turbulent flow in which resistance is proportional to gas density. Therefore, under conditions of laminar flow, the clinical use of a low-density, high-viscosity gas (e.g., helium) will do nothing to improve gas flow. However, if excessive airway resistance is caused by turbulence (as in croup or other forms of airway obstruction), density, not viscosity, becomes important.

Reynold's Number

The factors that determine whether flow in a tube will be laminar or turbulent are related in the equation that defines a dimensionless quantity called the Reynold's number:

$$N_R = \frac{\text{inertial force}}{\text{viscous force}} = \frac{\rho v^2}{\eta(v/2r)} = \frac{\rho 2 r v}{\eta}$$

where

v = average linear velocity of the gas (cm/s)

r = radius of tube (cm)

ρ = density of gas (g/cm^3)

η = viscosity in poise (dyne · s/cm^2)

In straight, smooth tubes, turbulence for most fluids is probable when the Reynold's number exceeds 2000. Once flow becomes turbulent, the pressure difference required to produce a given gas flow rate through a given passage is proportional to gas density and the square of the gas flow rate but is independent of viscosity.

Bernoulli Theorem

For an incompressible fluid in laminar flow (assuming that there are no energy losses from friction), Bernoulli's equation states that the energy densities at any two points in the system are equal:

$$PE_1 = P_1 + KE_1 = PE_2 + P_2 + KE_2$$

where

PE = potential energy per unit volume or height × density × gravitational acceleration

P = pressure of the gas measured perpendicular to flow

KE = kinetic energy per unit volume or 1/2 density × velocity squared

Consider a fluid that flows from a relatively wide section of tubing (subscript 1 in the above equation) to a relatively narrow section (subscript 2). Since the cross-sectional area in the narrow section is smaller, the velocity of the fluid must increase to keep the flow rate the same. As a result, the kinetic energy density (KE_2) increases. Assuming that the potential energy density stays the same, the pressure (P_2) at this point must decrease so that the right side of the equation remains equal to the left. Stated simply, as the forward velocity of the fluid increases, its radial pressure decreases. This is often called the Bernoulli effect.

Henry's Law (Law of Solubility)

When a liquid and gas are in equilibrium, the amount of gas in solution is directly proportional to the partial pressure of the gas if temperature is constant. Expressed mathematically this is

$$C = 0.132\alpha P$$

where

C = gas concentration in vol% (mL gas/dL liquid)

α = the Bunsen solubility coefficient of the gas (mL gas STPD/mL solvent) (see Table 4–2)

P = gas partial pressure (mm Hg)

0.132 = a constant equal to 100/760 used to express C in vol%

Table 4-2 Bunsen Solubility Coefficients (mL STPD/mL Solvent)[*]

Gas	Plasma	Blood[**]
He	0.0154	0.0149
N_2	0.0117	0.0130
O_2	0.0209	0.0240
CO_2	0.5100	0.4700

[*]Gas partial pressure = 760 mm Hg and temperature = 37°C.
[**]Hematocrit = 0.45.

Graham's Law (Law of Diffusion)

Graham's law states that the diffusion of a gas is inversely proportional to the square root of its molecular weight. For example, in comparing the relative rates of diffusion of carbon dioxide and oxygen, we get

$$\frac{D_{CO_2}}{D_{O_2}} = \frac{\sqrt{gmw\ O_2}}{\sqrt{gmw\ CO_2}} = \frac{\sqrt{32}}{\sqrt{44}} = \frac{5.6}{6.6}$$

where

D_{CO_2} = diffusion coefficient for carbon dioxide

D_{O_2} = diffusion coefficient for oxygen

gmw = gram molecular weight

From this we see that carbon dioxide diffuses only 0.85 times as fast as oxygen in the gaseous state owing to carbon dioxide's greater molecular weight.

Fick's Law of Diffusion

The factors controlling the rate of diffusion of a gas into or out of a liquid are expressed in the equation

$$\dot{V}GAS \propto \; = \frac{\Delta P \times A \times S}{d \times \sqrt{gmw}}$$

where

$\dot{V}GAS$ = diffused gas flow

ΔP = pressure gradient across the gas–liquid interface

A = cross-sectional area

S = solubility of gas

d = distance for diffusion

gmw = gram molecular weight of the gas

In comparing the rates of diffusion of carbon dioxide and oxygen through an aqueous medium, it should be noted that for the same *concentration* gradient, carbon dioxide diffuses more slowly than oxygen. However, because of its 25 times greater solubility, carbon dioxide diffuses 20 times faster than oxygen for the same *tension* gradient.

Law of Laplace (for a Sphere)

The pressure difference between the inside and outside of a sphere is dependent on the surface tension of the air–liquid interface and the radius of the bubble. For a sphere with one air–liquid interface (e.g., an alveolus or a gas bubble in a liquid), the equation is

$$PTRANS = \frac{2T}{r}$$

where

$PTRANS$ = transmural pressure differences (dyne/cm^2)

T = surface tension (dyne/cm)

r = radius of sphere (cm)

For a sphere with two air–liquid interfaces (e.g., a sphere of gas enclosed in a thin film of liquid such as a soap bubble), the equation becomes

$$PTRANS = \frac{4T}{r}$$

In either case, the Laplace equation indicates that the smaller the radius of the sphere, the higher its transmural pressure difference. Thus, it would seem that a small alveolus would have the natural tendency to empty its gas into a larger one and collapse. This tendency is counteracted by the presence of surfactant on the inner surface of the alveolus. Surfactant decreases the surface tension inside the alveolus in proportion to the ratio of surfactant to alveolar surface area. As an alveolus becomes smaller, the amount of surfactant per unit of surface area increases. This causes the surface tension to decrease to a greater extent than the corresponding reduction of radius so that the pressure ($= 2T/r$) decreases. Thus, small alveoli in communication with large alveoli are able to equilibrate to the same pressure without collapsing.

Absolute Humidity

Absolute humidity is the water vapor density expressed in grams per cubic meter (or milligrams per liter) of air. It can be estimated using the following equation (derived from the ideal gas equation):

$$\text{AH} = \frac{287.7 \times \text{RH} \times \text{P}_{\text{SAT}}}{t + 273}$$

where

AH = absolute humidity (mg/L or g/m^3)

RH = relative humidity expressed as a decimal

P_{SAT} = the partial pressure of saturated water vapor (mm Hg) at the given temperature, t

t = temperature (°C)

Relative Humidity

The ratio of the actual amount of water vapor in a gas (absolute humidity) at a given temperature to the amount of water vapor the gas could hold if saturated at that temperature (capacity) is the relative humidity. Mathematically, it is

$$\text{relative humidity } (\%) = \frac{\text{absolute humidity}}{\text{capacity}} \times 100$$

$$\text{relative humidity } (\%) = \frac{\text{measured water vapor pressure}}{\text{saturated water vapor pressure}} \times 100$$

Goff–Gratch Equation

Saturated water vapor pressure can be estimated from the temperature of the gas using the following adaptation of the Goff–Gratch equation (in computer or calculator notation):

$$\text{P\textsc{sat}} = K * (10\char`\^(((-7.90298) * (373.16/t - 1))$$
$$+ (5.02808 * \text{LOG}(373.16/t))$$
$$- (1.3816 * 10\char`\^(-7) * (10\char`\^(11.334 * (1 - t/373.16)) - 1))$$
$$+ (8.132 * 10\char`\^(-3) * (10\char`\^(-3.49149 * (373.16/t - 1)) - 1))))$$

where t is the temperature of the gas in degrees kelvin, LOG is logarithm (base 10), and K is a constant determined by the desired units for P\textsc{sat}. The symbol ∘ stands for multiplication, / stands for division, and ^ represents exponentiation (i.e., $10\char`\^2 = 100$). Table 4–3 gives the values of K for various units of pressure.

Table 4-3 Goff-Gratch Equation Constants for Various Units of Pressure

Desired Unit	K
atmosphere (atm)	1
pounds/in.^{2} (psi)	14.696
inches of mercury (in. Hg)	29.9213
millimeters of mercury (mm Hg)	760
centimeters of water (cm H_2O)	1033.26
millibars (mb)	1013.25
kilopascals (kPa)	101.3

Antoine Equation

The saturated vapor pressure of water and a variety of anesthetic gases can be estimated using the Antoine equation:

$$\text{P\textsc{sat}} = \text{antilog}\left(A - \frac{B}{t + C}\right)$$

where

P\textsc{sat} = units of pressure desired

antilog = the antilogarithm (base 10) of the expression in parentheses

A, B, and C = constants whose values depend on the chemical composition of the vapor. Table 4–4 gives values of A, B, and C for water and varieties of anesthetic gases.

t = temperature (°C)

Table 4-4 Antoine Equation Data

Substance	A (kPA) (mm Hg)	B	C	Temperature Range of Data (°C)	Maximum Deviation from Data
Water	7.16728 8.04343	1716.984	232.538	−5–135	1%
Nitrous oxide	6.70184 7.57799	912.8988	285.309	−40–36	1%
Halothane	5.89184 6.76799	1043.697	218.262	−51–55	3%
Isoflurane	4.82163 5.69778	536.4589	140.991	25–49	1%
Enflurane	6.11225 6.98840	1107.839	213.063	17–56	0.3%

Table 4–5 gives values for water vapor pressure, content, and saturation for temperatures, commonly encountered in health care.

Table 4-5 Water Vapor Pressure, Content, and Percent Saturation

Temperature (°C)	Vapor Pressure (mm Hg)	Water Content (mg/L)	% Saturation at 37°C
20	17.54	17.30	39
22	19.88	19.42	44
24	22.38	21.78	50
26	25.21	24.36	55
28	28.35	27.22	62
30	31.82	30.35	69
32	35.66	33.76	77
34	39.90	37.56	86

(continued)

Table 4-5 Water Vapor Pressure, Content, and Percent Saturation (continued)

Temperature (°C)	Vapor Pressure (mm Hg)	Water Content (mg/L)	% Saturation at 37°C
36	44.56	41.70	95
37	47.07	43.90	100
38	49.69	46.19	–
40	55.32	51.10	–
42	61.50	56.50	–

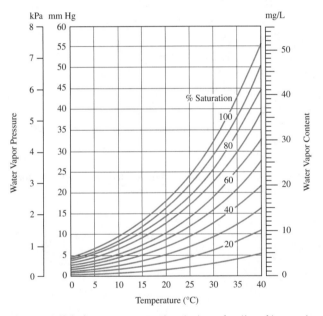

Figure 4-1 Water vapor pressure and content as a function of temperature (from the Antoine equation).

OXYGEN ADMINISTRATION

Blender or Entrainment System Equations

The following equations relate the variables of oxygen, flow, airflow, total flow, and fraction of inspired oxygen (FIO_2) when blenders or entrainment systems are used.

$$\text{FIO}_2 = \frac{O_2 \text{ flow} + (0.21 \times \text{ airflow})}{\text{total flow}}$$

$$= 0.21 + \frac{(0.79 \times O_2 \text{ flow})}{\text{total flow}}$$

$$O_2 \text{ flow} = \frac{\text{total flow} \times (\text{FIO}_2 - 0.21)}{0.79}$$

$$\text{airflow} = \text{total flow} - O_2 \text{ flow}$$

$$\text{total flow} = \frac{O_2 \text{ flow} \times 0.79}{\text{FIO}_2 - 0.21}$$

$$\frac{\text{airflow}}{O_2 \text{ flow}} = \frac{1.0 - \text{FIO}_2}{\text{FIO}_2 - 0.21}$$

These equations were derived from the general equations

$$(\text{FO}_2)(\text{total flow}) = (\text{FAO}_2)(\text{flow A}) + (\text{FBO}_2)(\text{flow B})$$

and

$$\text{total flow} = \text{flow A} + \text{flow B}$$

where

FO_2 = final fraction of oxygen in mixture

$\text{F}x\text{O}_2$ = fractional concentration of oxygen in the individual flows making up the mixture

This equation simply states that the total flow of oxygen in the mixture is equal to the sum of the flows of oxygen in the gases being blended together.

In the home care environment, it is often necessary to blend oxygen into the gas delivered by a home care ventilator, as these devices usually do not provide control of F_{IO_2}. If pure oxygen is used, the preceding equations apply. However, it may be convenient to use an oxygen concentrator. In this case, the fractional concentration of oxygen delivered by the concentrator (F_{CO_2}) must be known. The relationships among F_{IO_2} total minute ventilation ($\dot{V}_E$, the total flow of gas from the ventilator and the concentrator), concentrator flow rate ($\dot{V}_C$), and the flow of gas from the ventilator ($\dot{V}_{AIR}$ equal to the product of tidal volume and ventilator frequency) may be expressed as follows.

$$F_{IO_2} = \frac{\dot{V}_C \times F_{CO_2} + \dot{V}_{AIR} \times 0.21}{\dot{V}_E}$$

$$\dot{V}_E = \dot{V}_C \times \frac{F_{CO_2} - 0.21}{F_{IO_2} - 0.21}$$

$$\dot{V}_{AIR} = \dot{V}_C \times \frac{F_{CO_2} - F_{IO_2}}{F_{IO_2} - 0.21}$$

$$\dot{V}_{AIR} = \dot{V}_E - \dot{V}_E \times \frac{F_{IO_2} - 0.21}{F_{CO_2} - 0.21}$$

$$\dot{V}_C = \dot{V}_E \times \frac{F_{IO_2} - 0.21}{F_{CO_2} - 0.21}$$

If the F_{CO_2} drifts from its expected value due to concentrator malfunction, the resultant effect on F_{IO_2} may be estimated using the equation:

$$\text{act } F_{IO_2} = \frac{\text{expt } F_{IO_2} - 0.21}{\text{expt } F_{CO_2} - 0.21} \times (\text{act } F_{CO_2} - 0.21) + 0.21$$

where

    act = actual
    expt = expected

Derivation of Approximate F_{IO_2} for Low-Flow Oxygen System

$$F_{IO_2} = \text{volume of inspired } O_2 \div \text{tidal volume } (V_T)$$

volume of inspired O_2 = (a) volume of O_2 inspired from anatomic reservoir

plus

(b) volume of O_2 delivered by cannula during inspiration

plus

(c) volume of O_2 from inspired room air

Example

normal V_T = 500 mL

frequency = 20 breath/min

inspiratory time = 1 s

expiratory time = 2 s

period of no expiratory flow = 25% of expiratory time = 0.5 s

anatomic reservoir = 50 mL $\approx$ 30% of anatomic dead space

nasal cannula flow rate = 6 L/min (100 mL/s)

Thus,

(a) volume of O_2 inspired from anatomic reservoir = 100 mL/s × 0.5 s = 50 mL

(b) volume of O_2 delivered by cannula during inspiration = 100 mL/s × 1.0 s = 100 mL

(c) volume of O_2 from inspired room air = 0.20 × (V_T − V_D) = 0.20 × (500 − 150) = 70 mL

Therefore,

volume of inspired O_2 = 50 mL + 100 mL + 70 mL = 220 mL

and

$$F_{IO_2} = 220 \text{ mL} \div 500 \text{ mL} = 0.44$$

Table 4-6 Low-Flow Oxygen Systems[*]

System	O_2 Flow Rate (L/min)	Approximate F_{IO_2}
Nasal cannula or catheter	1	0.24
	2	0.28
	3	0.32
	4	0.36
	5	0.40
	6	0.44
Simple oxygen mask	5-10	0.35-0.50
Mask with reservoir bag	8-10	0.60-0.80

[*]Normal tidal volume and respiratory rate are assumed.
Data from Wilkins, R. L., Stoller, J. K., Kacmarek, R. M. Egan's Fundamentals of Respiratory Care. 9th Edition. St. Louis: Mosby Elsevier; 2009:874.

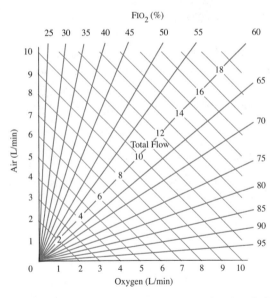

Figure 4-2 Inspired oxygen concentration as a function of mixed air and oxygen flow rates (low range of flow).

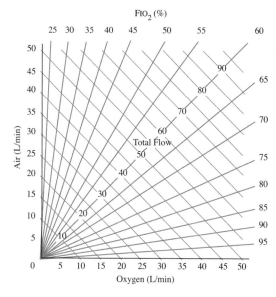

Figure 4-3 Inspired oxygen concentration as a function of mixed air and oxygen flow rates (high range of flow).

■ GAS CYLINDERS

Duration of Cylinders

The first step in calculating the duration of flow from a cylinder of compressed gas is to relate the decrease in cylinder volume to the drop in the cylinder's gauge pressure. The factor K, relating gas volume to pressure drop, is calculated as follows:

$$K \, (L/psi) \; = \; \frac{28.3 \, (L/ft^3) \times \; \text{volume of gas in full cylinder} \, (ft^3)}{\text{pressure of full cylinder (psi)}}$$

where

  28.3 = the factor to convert cubic feet to liters

Table 4–7 gives values for the K factors for different gases and cylinder sizes.

Once the value of K is found for a particular size of cylinder, the duration of constant flow can be calculated from the gauge pressure using the equation:

$$\text{duration of flow (min)} = \frac{K \times \text{gauge pressure (psi)}}{\text{flow rate (L/min)}}$$

Table 4–8 gives approximate number of hours of flow according to cylinder size.

Helium Therapy

Helium is odorless, tasteless, nonexplosive, and physiologically inert. Because of its low density, helium has been used in the management of airway obstruction where turbulent gas flow patterns cause an increase in airway resistance and increase the work of breathing. Commercially pre-pared cylinders of helium–oxygen mixtures are available in 80%–20% and 70%–30% combinations.

Because the calibration of standard flowmeters (i.e., Thorpe tube) depends on gas properties, a correction must be applied when helium–oxygen mixtures are used with flowmeters calibrated for oxygen or air. The *calibration* factor of a flowmeter is inversely proportional to the square root of the molecu-lar weight of the gas. Therefore, if a 70%–30% helium–oxygen mixture is used with an *oxygen* flowmeter, the measured flow must be multiplied by $\sqrt{\text{gmw O}_2}/\sqrt{\text{gmw mixture}}$ to obtain the actual flow rate. Thus, to obtain a desired flow rate of a given mixture with an oxygen flowmeter, the following equations are used.

80%–20% helium–oxygen mixture:

$$\text{required flowmeter setting} = \frac{\text{desired flow rate}}{1.8}$$

70%–30% helium–oxygen mixture:

$$\text{required flowmeter setting} = \frac{\text{desired flow rate}}{1.6}$$

Gas Therapy Working Tables and Figures

Table 4-7 K Factors (L/psi) to Calculate Duration of Cylinder Flow

Gas	Cylinder Size			
	D	E	G	H and K
O_2, CO_2, N_2, air	0.16	0.28	2.41	3.14
O_2/CO_2	0.20	0.35	2.94	3.84
He/O_2	0.14	0.23	1.93	2.50

Table 4-8 Approximate Number of Hours of Flow

Flow Rate (L/min)	Cylinder Type							
	Full		3/4 Full		1/2 Full		1/4 Full	
	E	H	E	H	E	H	E	H
2	5.1	56	3.8	42	2.5	28	1.3	14
4	2.	28	1.8	21	1.2	14	0.6	7
6	1.7	18.5	1.3	13.7	0.9	9.2	0.4	4.5
8	1.2	14	0.9	10.5	0.6	7	0.3	3.5
10	1.0	11	0.7	8.2	0.5	5.5	0.2	2.7
12	0.8	9.2	0.6	6.7	0.4	4.5	0.2	2.2
15	0.6	7.2	0.4	5.5	0.3	3.5	0.1	1.7

Table 4-9 Medical Gas Cylinder Color Codes*

Gas	Symbol	United States	International
Carbon dioxide	CO_2	Gray	Gray
Cyclopropane	C_3H_6	Orange	Orange
Ethylene	C_2H_6	Red	Violet
Helium	He	Brown	Brown
Nitrous oxide	N_2O	Blue	Blue
Oxygen	O_2	Green	White
Oxygen-carbon dioxide		Gray + green	Gray + white
Oxygen-helium		Brown + green	Brown + white
Air		Yellow + silver	White + black

*Note: Color codes are accurate for E cylinders only.

Table 4-10 Medical Gas Cylinder Dimensions

Size	Diameter (in.)	Diameter (cm)	Height (in.)	Height (cm)	Weight (lb)	Weight (kg)
A	3	7.6	10	25.4	2.5	5.5
B	3.5	8.9	16	40.6	5.25	11.6
D	4.25	10.8	20	50.8	10.25	22.6
E	4.5	11.4	30	76.2	15	33
M	7	17.8	47	119.4	66	145.2
G	8.5	21.6	55	139.7	98	215.6
H&K	9	22.9	55	139.7	100	220

Table 4-11 Medical Gas Cylinder Specifications

Gas	Pressure (psi)		Cylinder Size D	E	G	H & K
Oxygen	1800-2400	ft^3	12.6	22	186	244
		L	356	622	5260	6900
Carbon dioxide	840	ft^3	33	56	425	
		L	934	1585	12,000	
Helium	1650-2000	ft^3	10.6	17	146	
		L	300	480	4130	
Nitrous oxide	745	ft^3	34.5	57	485	577
		L	975	1610	13,750	15,800
Cyclopropane	80	ft^3	30			
		L	848			
Ethylene	1250	ft^3	26.6	44	372	
		L	752	1245	10,500	
Oxygen–carbon dioxide mix	1500-2200	ft^3	12.6	22	186	
		L	356	622	5620	
Oxygen–helium mix	1650-2000	ft^3	11	18	150	
		L	310	510	4250	

Table 4–12 Pin Index and CGA Standards

Gas	Pin Position	CGA Con. No.*
Oxygen	2-5	870
Carbon dioxide-oxygen (CO$_2$ not over 7%)	2-6	880
Helium-oxygen (He not over 80%)	2-4	890
Ethylene	1-3	900
Nitrous oxide	3-5	910
Cyclopropane	3-6	920
Helium	4-6	930
Helium-oxygen (He not over 80%)		
Carbon dioxide	1-6	940
Carbon dioxide-oxygen (CO$_2$ over 7%) (mixtures other than those shown above; for lab use only)	No CGA standard	

*CGA Con. = Compressed Gas Association connection.

Table 4–13 New Standard Threaded Valve Outlet Connections for Medical Gases

Gas	Outlet Thread	CGA Connection
Oxygen	0.903"-14NGO-RH-EXT.	540
Carbon dioxide		
Carbon dioxide-oxygen (CO$_2$ over 7%)	0.825"-14NGO-RH-EXT. (flat nipple)	320
Carbon dioxide-oxygen (CO$_2$ not over 7%)		
Helium-oxygen (He not over 80%)	0.745"-14NGO-RH-EXT.	280
Helium		
Helium-oxygen (He over 80%)	0.965"-14NGO-RH-INT.	580
Nitrous oxide	0.825"-14NGO-RH-EXT. (small round nipple)	1320
Ethylene	0.825"-14NGO-LH-EXT. (round nipple)	350
Cyclopropane	0.885"-14NGO-LH-INT.	510
Special mixtures (mixtures other than those shown above)	0.825"-14NGO-RH-EXT. (flat nipple)	320

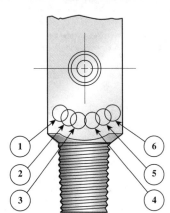

Figure 4-4 PPLT index, CGA standard. (See Table 4-12.)

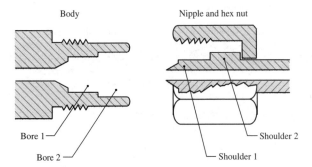

Figure 4-5 Schematic illustration of components of a representative diameter index safety system (DISS) connection. The two shoulders of the nipple allow the nipple to unite only with a body having corresponding borings.

Table 4–14 Gas Volume Correction Equations*

To Convert From	To	Multiply By
ATPS (ambient temperature and pressure, saturated with water vapor)	STPD	$\dfrac{P_B - P_{H_2O}}{760} \times \dfrac{273}{273 + T}$
	BTPS	$\dfrac{P_B - P_{H_2O}}{P_B - 47} \times \dfrac{310}{273 + T}$
	ATPD	$\dfrac{P_B - P_{H_2O}}{P_B}$
ATPD (ambient temperature and pressure, dry)	STPD	$\dfrac{P_B}{760} \times \dfrac{273}{273 + T}$
	BTPS	$\dfrac{P_B}{P_B - 47} \times \dfrac{310}{273 + T}$
	ATPS	$\dfrac{P_B}{P_B - P_{H_2O}}$
BTPS (body temperature and ambient pressure, saturated with water vapor at body temperature)	STPD	$\dfrac{P_B - 47}{760} \times \dfrac{273}{310}$
	ATPS	$\dfrac{P_B - 47}{P_B - P_{H_2O}} \times \dfrac{273 + T}{310}$
	ATPD	$\dfrac{P_B - 47}{P_B} \times \dfrac{273 + T}{310}$
STPD (standard temperature and pressure, dry)	BTPS	$\dfrac{760}{P_B - 47} \times \dfrac{310}{273}$
	ATPS	$\dfrac{760}{P_B - P_{H_2O}} \times \dfrac{273 + T}{273}$
	ATPD	$\dfrac{760}{P_B} \times \dfrac{273 + T}{273}$

*Based on ambient temperature (T) in °C, barometric pressure (P_B) in mm Hg, and the saturating pressure of water (P_{H_2O}) in mm Hg at ambient temperature.

Table 4-15 Conversion Factors to Correct Volume (ATPS) to Volume (BTPS)*

Gas Temperature (°C)	Factor
20	1.102
21	1.096
22	1.091
23	1.085
24	1.080
25	1.075
26	1.068
27	1.063
28	1.057
29	1.051
30	1.045
31	1.039
32	1.032
33	1.026
34	1.020
35	1.014
36	1.007
37	1.000

*Volume (BTPS) = volume (ATPS) × conversion factor.
Note: These factors have been calculated for a barometric pressure of 760 mm Hg. Small deviations from standard barometric pressure have little effect on the correction factors (e.g., the factor for gas at 22°C and 770 mm Hg is 1.0904).

Table 4-16 Physical Characteristics of Gases

Gas	Density (g/L)	Critical Temperature (°C)	Critical Pressure (psi)	Boiling Point (°C)	Melting Point (°C)
Air	1.29	−140.7	546.8	–	–
Oxygen	1.43	−118.8	730.6	−182.9	−218.4
Carbon dioxide	1.97	31.1	1,073.1	−78.5 (sublimates)	−56.6 (at 5.2 atm)
Nitrogen	1.25	−147.1	492.5	−195.8	−209.9

Table 4-17 Effects of Breathing Oxygen During Hyperbaric Therapy

	Air (at 1 atm)	Oxygen (at 1 atm)	Oxygen (at 3 atm)
Hemoglobin concentration	0.15 kg/L	0.15 kg/L	0.15 kg/L
Oxyhemoglobin	200 mL	204 mL	204 mL
Dissolved oxygen	2.85 mL/L	13.5 mL/L	42.3 mL/L
Total oxygen	203 mL/L	217 mL/L	246 mL/L

Table 4-18 Atmospheric Content, Percent by Volume

Nitrogen	78.084
Oxygen	20.947
Water	0.750
Carbon dioxide	0.031

CHAPTER

5

Mechanical Ventilation

This chapter brings together a large variety of information concerning the equipment and theory of mechanical ventilation. Some of the material has been gathered from the manufacturers' data sheets. We have attempted to present the data in a uniform structure for easy comparison.

■ AIRWAYS

Table 5-1 Dimensions of Oral Airways

Age	ISO Size	Length (mm)	Guedel	Berman
Neonate	4	40	Pink	Pink
Infant	5	50	Blue	Turquoise
Small child	6	60	Black	Black
Child	7	70	White	White
Small adult	8	80	Green	Green
Medium adult	9	90	Yellow	Yellow
Adult	10	100	Red	Purple
Large adult	11	110	Orange	Orange

Table 5-2 Approximate Equivalents of Various Tracheostomy Tube

Jackson Size	Outside Diameter (mm)	French	Internal Diameter (mm)
00	4.3	13	2.5
0	5.0	15	3.0
1	5.5	16.5	3.5
2	6.0	18	4.0
3	7	21	4.5-5.0
4	8	24	5.5
5	9	27	6.0-6.5
6	10	30	7.0
7	11	33	75-8.0
8	12	37	8.5
9	13	39	9.0-9.5
10	14	42	10.0
11	15	45	10.5-11.0
12	16	48	11.5

Note: Since tube thicknesses vary from one manufacturer to another, these data are intended as a guide only.

Table 5-3 Dimensions of Cuffless Pediatric Tracheostomy Tubes (in millimeters)

Size	ID	OD	L
Portex			
2.5	2.5	4.5	30
3.0	3.0	5.2	36
3.5	3.5	5.8	40
4.0	4.0	6.6	44
4.5	4.5	7.1	48
Shiley			
3.0	3.0	4.5	39
3.5	3.5	5.2	40
4.0	4.0	6.0	41
4.5	4.5	6.5	42
5.0	5.0	7.1	44

ID = internal diameter; OD = outside diameter; L = length.

Table 5-4 Dimensions of Low-Pressure Cuffed Adult Tracheostomy Tubes (in millimeters)

Size	ID	OD	L
Kamen-Wilkenson (Bivona) (Fome-Cuff)			
5	5.0	7.3	60
6	6.0	8.7	70
7	7.0	10	80
8	8.0	11	88
9	9.0	12.3	98
Portex			
6	6.0	8.3	55
7	7.0	9.7	75
8	8.0	11	82
9	9.0	12.4	87

Table 5-4 Dimensions of Low-Pressure Cuffed Adult Tracheostomy Tubes (in millimeters) (continued)

Size	ID	OD	L
Shiley			
4	5.0	9.4	65
6	6.4	10.8	76
8	7.5	12.2	81
10	8.9	13.8	81

ID = internal diameter; OD = outside diameter; L = length.

Table 5-5 Laryngoscope Blades

	Miller		Wisconsin		Macintosh	
Age	Size	Length (mm)	Size	Length (mm)	Size	Length (mm)
Premature infant	0	75	0	75	–	–
Infant	1	102	1	102	1	91
Child	2	150	2	135	2	100
Adult	3	190	3	162	3	130
Large adult	–	–	4	199	4	190

Table 5-6 Approximate Equivalents of Various Endotracheal Tube Sizing Methods[*]

Diameter Sizing					Equivalent Connector Size (mm)
Internal (mm)	External (mm)	Magill Gauge	French Gauge	Equivalent Cuffs (in.)	
2.5	4.0		12		3
3.0	4.5	00	12-14		
3.5	5.0	0-0	14-16	3/16	4
4.0	5.5	0-1	16-18	3/16	
4.5	6.0	1-2	18-20	1/4	5
5.0	6.5	1-2	20-22	1/4	
5.5	7.0	3-4	22	1/4	6
6.0	8.0	3-4	24	1/4	
6.5	8.5	4-5	26	1/4	7

Table 5-6 Approximate Equivalents of Various Endotracheal Tube Sizing Methods[*] (continued)

Diameter Sizing					Equivalent Connector Size (mm)
Internal (mm)	External (mm)	Magill Gauge	French Gauge	Equivalent Cuffs (in.)	
7.0	9.0	5-6	28	5/16	
7.5	9.5	6-7	30	5/16	8
8.0	10.0	7-8	32	5/16	9
8.5	11.5	8	34	3/8	
9.0	12.0	9-10	36	3/8	10
9.5	12.5	9-10	38	3/8	11
10.0	13.0	10-11	40	7/16	12
10.5	13.5	10-11	42	7/16	
11.0	14.5	11-12	42-44	1/2	13
11.5	15.0	11-12	44-46	1/2	

[*]Since tube thicknesses vary from one manufacturer to another, these data are intended as a guide only.

Table 5-7 Guide to Choice of Endotracheal Tubes[*]

	French Size	Internal Diameter (mm)	Oral Length (cm)	Nasal Length (cm)	Suction Catheter (French)
<1000 g	12	2.5	8	11	6
≥1000 g	14	3.0	9	12	6
6 mo	16	3.5	10	14	8
1 yr	18-20	4.0-4.5	12	16	8
2 yr	22-24	5.0-5.5	14	17	8
2-4 yr	24-26	5.5-6.0	15	18	10
4-7 yr	26-28	6.0-6.5	16	19	10
7-10 yr	28-30	6.5-7.0	17	21	10
10-12 yr	30-32	7.0-7.5	20	23	10
12-16 yr	32-34	7.5-8.0	21	24	12
Adult (female)	34-36	8.0-8.5	22	25	12
Adult (male)	36-38	8.5-9.0	22	25	14

[*]Endotracheal tube sizes will vary with body size and height. One size smaller and one size larger should be available for individual variations.

Table 5-8 Appropriate Suction Settings Vacuum Settings

Vacuum Settings		
Age	Portable (in. Hg)	Wall (mm Hg)
Infant	3-5	60-100
Child	5-10	100-120
Adult	7-15	120-150

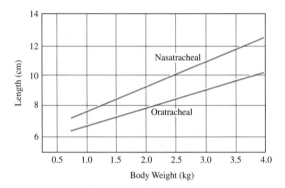

Figure 5-1 Graph for determining the appropriate length of insertion for infant endo-tracheal tubes. For infants weighing < 750 grams subtract 0.5 cm from predicted length.

Endotracheal (ET) tube size may be estimated for 1 to 12-year-olds by

$$\text{internal diameter of ET tube (mm)} = \frac{\text{age (yr)} + 16}{4}$$

■ DEFINITION OF TERMS

Note: In Tables 5–9a, 5–9b, and 5–9c and Figures 5–2 and 5–3, the use of italics and subscripts differs from the symbol notation style used in this book.

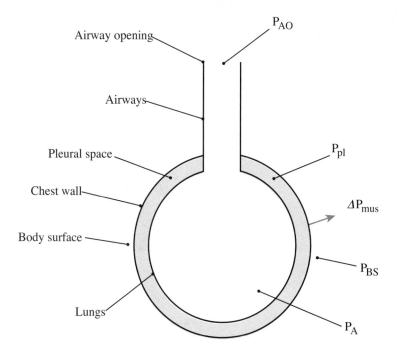

Figure 5-2 Schematic representation of the respiratory system, consisting of a flow conducting tube (representing the airways) connected to a single elastic compartment representing the lungs, surrounded by another elastic compartment representing the chest wall. P_{AO} is the pressure at the airway opening, P_{PL} is pressure in the intrapleural space, P_{BS} is pressure on the body surface, P_A is alveolar pressure, and $\Delta Pmus$ is muscle pressure difference.

Reprinted with permission from *Respir Care* 51(12) (2006), 1458-1470.

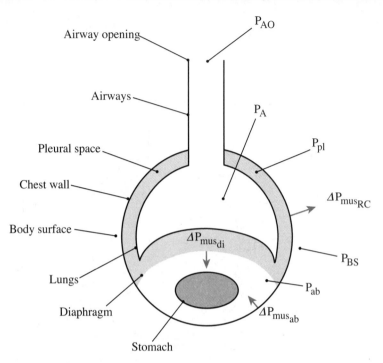

Figure 5-3 Diagram of the respiratory system with one compartment lung(s) and chest wall subdivided into rib cage, diapgragmatic, and abdominal wall components. The arrows labeled ΔPmus indicate the positive directions for the corresponding muscle pressure differences. P_{AO} = pressure at the airway opening. P_A = alveolar pressure. P_{pl} = pressure in the intrapleural space. ΔPmus = muscle pressure difference. RC = rib cage. BS = body surface. ab = abdomen. di = diaphragm.

Reprinted with permission from *Respir Care* 51(12) (2006), 1458-1470.

Table 5-9A Summary of Symbol Conventions

Entity	Subtype	Style	Examples	
Variable	Primary	Italic, upper case	P	pressure
			V	volume
			$\dot{V}$	flow
			C	concentration
			T	temperature
	Difference (difference between points in space)	Italic, upper case, delta symbol	ΔP	pressure at one point minus pressure at another point on the system
	Change (change relative to a reference point)	Italic, lower case	p	pressure measured relative to an operating point
Argument (used with variables only; if no argument explicitly stated, then time is implied)	Not applicable	Style of entity	$P(t)$	pressure as a function of time
			$v(p)$	change in volume as a function of change in pressure
			$\mathbf{Z}(j\omega)$	impedance (complex number; function of angular frequency)
Property	Material	Bold, usually Greek	$\boldsymbol{\varepsilon}$	elasticity
			$\boldsymbol{\eta}$	viscosity
	Structural	Bold, usually English	$\mathbf{C}$	compliance
			$\mathbf{R}$	resistance
			$\boldsymbol{\tau}$	time constant
			$\mathbf{I}$	inertance
			$\mathbf{D}$	diffusing capacity
	System	Bold, upper case may be English and Greek	$\mathbf{Z}(j\omega)$	impedance (complex number; function of angular frequency)
Characteristic	General waveform	Upper and lower case	PEEP	positive end expiratory pressure
			MAP	mean arterial pressure
			WOB	work of breathing
			PIP	peak inspiratory pressure
	System response	Upper and lower case	FEV_1	forced expiratory volume in the first second
			MV	minute ventilation
			FVC	forced vital capacity
			$\mathbf{C}$dyn	dynamic compliance

Reprinted with permission from *Respir Care* 51(12) (2006), 1458-1470.

Table 5-9B Summary of Symbol Modifier Conventions*

Entity	Subtype	Style	Examples	Entity
Modifier (note that modifier takes on the style of the entity it modifies)	Substance	Superscript	P^{O_2}	partial pressure o oxygen
	Location/direction	Subscript	$\bar{P}_{AO}$	mean pressure at airway opening
			$\mathbf{R}_{aw}$	resistance of the airways
			$P^{O_2}_a$	partial pressure (gauge) of oxygen in arterial blood
			$\dot{V}^{(t)}_E$	expiratory flow (here expressed as an explicit function of time)
	Time index	Subscript	$P_{0.1}$	occlusion pressure at 0.1 second after start of inspiration
			FEV_1	forced expiratory volume in the first second
			t_I	inspiratory time interval
			t_E	expiratory time interval
			τ	time constant
			$\Delta P_{TR,I}$	transrespiratory pressure difference at time I
	Descriptor (inherent part of name)	Small letters (not subscripted)	C_{dyn}	dynamic compliance
			V_D	dead space volume
			V_T	tidal volume

*Symbols over entities such as bars, dots, or double dots are normal mathematical conventions.
Reprinted with permission from *Respir Care* 51(12) (2006), 1458-1470.

Table 5-9C

Some Measurable Pressures Used in Describing Respiratory System Mechanics

Name	Symbol	Definition
Pressure at the airway opening	P_{AO}	Pressure measured at the opening of the respiratory system airway (eg, mouth/nose, tracheostomy opening, or end of endotracheal tube)
Pleural pressure	P_{pl}	Pressure measured in the pleural space; changes in pleural pressure are often estimated by measuring pressure changes in the esophagus
Alveolar pressure	P_A	Pressure in the alveolar (gas space) region of the lungs
Body surface pressure	P_{BS}	Pressure measured at the body surface
Abdominal pressure	P_{ab}	Pressure inside the abdomen

Some Pressure Differences Used in Describing Respiratory System Mechanics

Definition*	Name	Symbol
P_{AO}-P_{BS}	Transrespiratory pressure difference	ΔP_{TR}
P_{AO}-P_A	Transairway pressure difference	ΔP_{TAW}
P_{AO}-P_{pl}	Transpulmonary pressure difference	ΔP_{TP}
P_A-P_{pl}	Transalveolar pressure difference	ΔP_{TA}
P_A-P_{BS}	Transthoracic pressure difference	ΔP_{TT}
P_{pl}-P_{BS}	Transchest-wall pressure difference	ΔP_{TCW}
P_{pl}-P_{ab}	Transdiaphramatic pressure difference	ΔP_{TR}
P_{ab}-P_{BS}	Transabdominal-wall pressure difference	ΔP_{TabW}
Theoretical transmural (ribcase, abdominal wall, diaphragm, chest wall) pressure differences that would produce movements identical to those produced by the ventilatory muscles during breathing maneuvers	Rib cage muscle pressure difference	$\Delta P_{mus_{RC}}$
	Abdominal muscle pressure difference	$\Delta P_{mus_{ab}}$
	Diaphragmatic muscle pressure difference	$\Delta P_{mus_{di}}$
	Chest wall muscle pressure difference (chest wall includes rib cage, abdomen, and diaphragm)	$\Delta P_{mus_{CW}}$

*Terms are defined as in Tables 1 and 2.

Reprinted with permission from *Respir Care* 51(12) (2006), 1458-1470.

Alveolar Ventilation ($\dot{V}A$)

The cumulative volume of fresh gas entering the gas-exchanging portion of the lungs (respiratory bronchioles and alveoli) per minute. Alveolar ventilation is calculated as

$$\dot{V}A = (V_T - V_D) \times f_b$$

where

$\dot{V}A$ = alveolar ventilation (L/min)

V_T = tidal volume (L)

V_D = dead space volume (L)

f_b = breathing frequency (breaths/min)

Compliance

A property that describes the elastic behavior of a structure. It quantifies the volume change that results from a change in pressure difference across a system *at rest.* Compliance can be calculated as the ratio of the change in volume to the change in pressure difference occurring between instants in which the system is completely *at rest:*

$$C = \frac{\Delta V}{\Delta(P_I - P_O)} \tag{5–1}$$

where

C = compliance (L/cm H_2O)

ΔV = change in volume (L)

P_I = pressure inside the system

P_O = pressure on the outside surface of the system

Note: The symbol Δ indicates a change in the variable within the parentheses.

The system for which compliance is evaluated is defined by the points between which the pressure is measured. For example, we can evaluate the compliance of the physiologic system, which comprises the lungs and chest wall. The compliance of the lung is defined as

$$C_L = \frac{\Delta V_L}{\Delta(P_{AO} - P_{PL})} \tag{5–2}$$

where

C_L = lung compliance (L/cm H_2O)

ΔV_L = the change in lung volume (L)

P_{AO} = pressure at the airway opening (cm H_2O)

P_{PL} = intrapleural pressure (cm H_2O) (Clinically, changes in P_{PL} are estimated from changes in esophageal pressure.)

For the chest wall, the equation is

$$C_W = \frac{\Delta V_W}{\Delta(P_{PL} - P_{BS})} \tag{5–3}$$

where

C_W = chest wall compliance (L/cm H_2O)

ΔV_W = the change in the volume of the thoracic cavity (equal to V_L if there is no pneumothorax)

P_{BS} = pressure at the body surface (cm H_2O)

Also,

$$C_{RS} = \frac{\Delta V_L}{\Delta(P_{AO} - P_{BS})} \qquad (5\text{--}4)$$

where

C_{RS} = total respiratory system compliance (L/cm H_2O)

Equations (5–2), (5–3), and (5–4) can be combined to show that

$$\frac{1}{C_{RS}} = \frac{1}{C_L} + \frac{1}{C_W}$$

or

$$C_{RS} = \frac{C_L \times C_W}{C_L + C_W}$$

Another system for which a knowledge of compliance is useful is the ventilator circuit attached to the patient's airway. We can compute this patient circuit compliance as

$$C_{PC} = \frac{\text{tidal volume}}{\Delta(P_{AO} - P_{BS})} = \frac{\text{tidal volume}}{PIP - PEEP}$$

where

C_{PC} = patient circuit compliance

$(P_{AO} - P_{BS})$ = the difference between pressure at the airway opening and pressure on the body surface, with the patient connection port occluded

PIP = peak inspiratory pressure with patient connection port occluded

$PEEP$ = positive end-expiratory pressure (if any) with patient connection port occluded

Compliance evaluated by equations (5–1) to (5–4) is referred to as *static compliance* in the literature. In practice, the equations are sometimes applied to the respiratory system during breathing, and the variables V and P are measured at instants when the flow at the airway opening is zero rather than when the system is at rest. Compliance calculated in this way is called *dynamic compliance.*

Static and dynamic compliances are given various symbols: For static compliance we shall use C; for dynamic compliance we shall use $Cdyn(f_b)$, in which f_b indicates that Cdyn is evaluated at particular breathing frequencies. If equation (5–2) is evaluated for the lungs when they are completely at rest (C_L) and during breathing at different frequencies ($CdynL(f_b)$), and if the values obtained under both sets of conditions are the same (within 20%), then we can infer that the lungs have a uniform distribution of mechanical time constants. Such lungs can therefore be characterized by a single compliance (C_L) and a single resistance (R_L) at all breathing frequencies.

If $CdynL(f_b)$ and C_L are not equal at all frequencies (i.e., $Cdyn(f_b)$ decreases as f_b increases), then the lungs have a nonuniform distribution of mechanical time constants (i.e., different regions of the lungs have different products of local flow resistance and local static compliance). In this case $CdynL(f_b)$ describes the elastic load presented by the system at a particular breathing frequency and reflects both the resistances and compliances of all the lung regions.

During mechanical ventilation, static respiratory system compliance can be evaluated using the equation

$$C_{RS} = \frac{V_T}{P_{PLT} - PEEP}$$

where

C_{RS} = static respiratory system compliance (L/cm H_2O)

V_T = tidal volume delivered to patient (L)

P_{PLT} = proximal airway plateau pressure (cm H_2O)

PEEP = positive end-expiratory pressure in the lungs (cm H_2O)

Another index, the dynamic characteristic, is often confused with dynamic compliance:

$$\text{dynamic characteristic} = \frac{V_T}{PIP - PEEP}$$

where PIP is peak inspiratory pressure. This index is not compliance because the pressure change has a component due to airway resistance (i.e., PIP occurs while flow is still being delivered to the airway opening). For a given tidal volume and inspiratory flow rate, the dynamic characteristic will decrease as either airway resistance increases or compliance decreases. It should be interpreted as an index of the load experienced by the ventilator.

Compressor

A device whose internal volume can be changed to increase the pressure of the gas it contains. In mechanical ventilation, a compressor is the device primarily responsible for generating the pressure necessary to force gas into the patient's lungs.

Cycle

To cycle the ventilator means to terminate the inspiratory phase.

Dead Space Volume (VD)

Dead space volume is the respired gas volume that does not participate in gas exchange. This volume is commonly referred to as *physiologic dead space.* One component of the physiologic dead space can be identified with the conducting (non-gas-exchanging) airways extending from the upper airway to the respiratory bronchioles. This component is called the *anatomic dead space.* Normal physiologic dead space volume is roughly estimated as 2 mL/kg (1 mL/lb) of ideal body weight.

Duty Cycle

A term applied to a device that functions intermittently rather than continuously. It refers to the ratio of the time that a device operates to its total cycle time expressed as a percent (e.g., the "% inspiration" of the Siemens Servo *i* Ventilator). As it applies to mechanical ventilators, the duty cycle can be defined as

$$\text{duty cycle (\%)} = \frac{f \times T_I}{60} \times 100\% = \frac{T_I}{TCT} \times 100\% = \frac{I}{I + E} \times 100\%$$

and

$$\frac{I}{E} = \frac{\text{duty cycle}}{100\% - \text{duty cycle}}$$

where

$\quad$ f = ventilator frequency (breaths/min)

$\quad$ TI = inspiratory time (s)

$\quad$ TCT = total cycle time, or time for one ventilatory cycle of one inspiration and one expiration (s)

$\quad$ I = numerator of inspiratory:expiratory ratio

$\quad$ E = denominator of inspiratory:expiratory ratio

Elastance (E)

The reciprocal of compliance (C):

$$E = \frac{1}{C}$$

Equation of Motion

The respiratory system can be modeled as a single flow-conducting tube connected in series to a single elastic compartment (referred to as a single compartment model). The equation that relates pressure, volume, and flow (all of which are functions of time) for this model is called the *equation of motion.* One version of this equation is

During Inspiration:

$$P_{MUS} + P_{TR} = (E_{TR} \times V) + (R_{TR} \times \dot{V}) + aPEEP$$

$$= \frac{V}{C_{RS}} + (R_{RS} \times \dot{V}) + aPEEP$$

During Expiration when P_{MUS} and P_{TR} = 0:

$$(E_{RS} \times V) + aPEEP = -(R_{RS} \times \dot{V})$$

where

$\quad$ aPEEP = auto PEEP, equal to end-expiratory alveolar pressure minus set PEEP

$\quad$ P_{MUS} = the effective pressure difference generated by the respiratory muscles

$\quad$ P_{TR} = the change in transrespiratory system pressure (e.g., the pressure generated by a mechanical ventilator) measured relative to end-expiratory pressure

CRS = compliance of the respiratory system

V = volume change measured relative to end-expiratory volume (i.e., functional residual capacity [FRC])

RRS = resistance of the respiratory system

$\dot{V}$ = change in flow measured relative to end-expiration (i.e., relative to zero flow)

ERS = elastance of the respiratory system

The system described by the equation of motion is defined by the points in space between which the pressure difference is measured. Thus, the respiratory system (along with respiratory system compliance and resistance) is defined in terms of transrespiratory pressure (pressure at the airway opening minus pressure at the body surface); the lungs (along with lung compliance and resistance) are defined in terms of transpulmonary pressure (pressure at the airway opening minus pressure in the pleural space); and the chest wall (along with chest wall compliance and resistance) is defined in terms of transmural pressure (pressure in the pleural space minus pressure at the body surface). The equation of motion may also be expressed using transpulmonary pressure (with lung compliance and resistance) or transmural pressure (with chest wall compliance and resistance).

Expiratory Time (TE)

The time interval from the start of expiratory flow to the start of inspiratory flow. Expiratory time is the total cycle time minus the inspiratory time. For volume-limited, constant-flow ventilators, TE may be calculated from the following equation (assuming there is no inspiratory hold):

$$TE = TI - TE = \frac{60}{f} - \frac{VT}{\dot{V}I}$$

where

TE = expiratory time (s)

TI = inspiratory time (s)

TCT = total cycle time (s)

f = ventilatory frequency (breaths/min)

VT = tidal volume (L)

$\dot{V}I$ = inspiratory flow rate (L/s)

If the I:E ratio is known, T_E is calculated as

$$T_E = \frac{TCT \times E}{I + E} = \frac{60 \times E}{f \times (I + E)}$$

where

T_E = expiratory time (s)

TCT = total cycle time (s)

I = numerator of I:E ratio

E = denominator of I:E ratio

f = ventilatory frequency (breaths/min)

Frequency, Breathing (f_b)

The number of breathing cycles or breaths per unit time (usually minutes) produced spontaneously or initiated by the patient or by the ventilator.

Frequency, Ventilator (f)

Breathing cycles or breaths per unit time (usually minutes) produced by a ventilator.

Frequency, Ventilator (as related to gas exchange)

During volume-limited, controlled ventilation, the arterial carbon dioxide tension (Pa_{CO_2}) can be controlled by the ventilator frequency, since Pa_{CO_2} is inversely proportional to alveolar ventilation. Assuming steady state and the body's metabolic production of carbon dioxide remains constant, the ventilator frequency required to effect a desired Pa_{CO_2} is given by

new f = old f × (old V_A / new V_A) × (old Pa_{CO_2} / new Pa_{CO_2})

where

V_A = alveolar volume = tidal volume minus dead space volume

For example, suppose a ventilator frequency of 10 bpm results in a Pa_{CO_2} of 60 mm Hg, and a Pa_{CO_2} of 40 mm Hg is desired without making a change in V_T, then

new f = 10 × 1 × 60/40 = 15 breaths/min

Gauge Pressure

Gauge pressure is the difference between the pressure of a fluid at some point and atmospheric pressure. Gauge pressure is denoted by a lower case g (e.g., psig or cm H_2O, g).

Inspiration

The act of inflating the lungs. Inspiration only occurs while there is flow into the airway opening.

Inspiratory:Expiratory Time Ratio (I:E)

Ratio of the inspiratory time to the expiratory time:

$$I:E = I/E$$

In the above equation, I and E can be expressed using either of the following conventions:

$$I = T_I/T_E \quad \text{(for example, 2:1)}$$
$$E = 1$$

or

$$I = 1$$
$$E = T_E/T_I, \quad \text{(for example, 1:3, 1:0.5)}$$

where

T_I = inspiratory time
T_E = expiratory time

Inspiratory Flow ($\dot{V}_I$)

The flow of gas measured at the airway opening during inspiration. For volume control modes, mean inspiratory flow rate can be calculated as

$$\dot{V}_I = \frac{V_T}{T_I}$$

where

$\dot{V}_I$ = inspiratory flow (L/min)
V_T = tidal volume (L)
T_I = inspiratory time (min)

Inspiratory Hold

A maneuver used during mechanical ventilation. It is characterized by a delay between the end of inspiratory flow and the beginning of expiratory flow. This delay period extends the inspiratory time.

Inspiratory Time (TI)

The time interval from the start of inspiratory flow to the start of expiratory flow. Note that TI can extend beyond the point when inspiration ends as when an inspiratory hold is used. Inspiratory time is equal to the total cycle time (TCT) minus the expiratory time. For volume-limited constant flow ventilators, TI may be calculated from the following equation (assuming there is no inspiratory hold):

$$T_I = \frac{V_T}{\dot{V}_I}$$

where

T_I = inspiratory time (s)

V_T = tidal volume (L)

$\dot{V}_I$ = inspiratory flow (L/s)

If the I/E ratio is known, TI is given by

$$T_I = \frac{TCT \times I}{I + E} = \frac{60 \times I}{f \times (I + E)}$$

where

T_I = inspiratory time (s)

TCT = total cycle time (s)

I = numerator of I:E ratio

E = denominator of I:E ratio

f = ventilatory frequency (breaths/min)

Inspiratory Relief Valve

A unidirectional valve designed to admit air to the patient system when the patient inspires spontaneously and the supply of inspiratory gases from the ventilator is inadequate.

Inspiratory Triggering Flow (V̇TR)

The flow that must be generated by the patient at the patient connection port to produce a drop in pressure (i.e., below the inspiratory triggering pressure) sufficient to initiate the ventilator inspiratory phase.

Inspiratory Triggering Pressure (PTR)

The airway pressure at the patient connection port that must be generated by the patient to initiate the ventilator inspiratory phase.

Inspiratory Triggering Response Time (TTR)

Time delay between the satisfaction of the inspiratory triggering pressure, flow, or volume requirements and the start of inspiratory flow.

Inspiratory Triggering Volume (VTR)

The volume change of the patient system plus the patient's lungs required to initiate the ventilator inspiratory phase.

Maximum Safety Pressure (PS MAX)

The highest gauge pressure that can be attained in the patient system during malfunction of the ventilator, but with functioning safety mechanisms (i.e., the valve opens).

Maximum Working Pressure (PW MAX)

The highest gauge pressure that can be attained in the patient system during the inspiratory phase when the ventilator is functioning normally. (This may be limited by ventilator adjustments to less than PS MAX.)

Mean Airway Pressure (P̄aw)

The average pressure that exists in the airways over a given integral number of cycles during mechanical ventilation. For a periodic waveform, P̄aw is defined as

$$\bar{P}aw = \frac{\text{area under pressure curve for one cycle}}{\text{total cycle time}}$$

In general,

$$\overline{Paw} = \frac{k(PIP - PEEP) \times TI}{TCT} + PEEP$$

where

Paw = mean airway pressure (cm H_2O)

k = waveform constant. The value of k depends on the shape of the airway pressure curve.

PIP = peak inspiratory pressure (cm H_2O)

$PEEP$ = positive end-expiratory pressure (cm H_2O)

TI = inspiratory time (sec)

TCT = total cycle time (sec)

For a constant flow ventilator with a periodic triangular pressure waveform and negligible expiratory resistance, the value of k in the preceding equation is $\frac{1}{2}$. For a periodic rectangular pressure waveform, the value of k is 1.0.

Minimum Safety Pressure (Ps MIN)

The most negative gauge pressure that can be attained in the patient system during malfunction of the ventilator, but with functioning safety mechanisms.

Minimum Working Pressure (Pw MIN)

The most negative gauge pressure that can be attained in the patient system during the expiratory phase when the ventilator is functioning normally. (This may be limited by ventilator adjustment to a pressure that is greater than Ps MIN.)

Minute Volume ($\dot{V}E$; Also, Minute Ventilation)

The cumulative volume of gas expired per minute by the patient:

$$\dot{V}E = VT \times f$$

where

$\dot{V}E$ = minute volume (L/min)

VT = tidal volume (L)

f = ventilatory frequency (breaths/min)

Motor

Anything that produces motion. As it relates to a mechanical ventilator, the motor is the device used to drive the compressor.

Patient System

That part of the ventilator gas system (up to the patient connection point) through which respired gas travels at respiratory pressures.

Pendelluft

Gas flow between different regions of the lung caused by inequalities of mechanical time constants among these regions.

Plateau Pressure (PPLT)

That portion of the proximal airway pressure waveform generated during positive pressure ventilation that is due solely to the elastic recoil of the total respiratory system (chest wall plus lungs). During volume-limited ventilation, this pressure is generated in the lung by delivering a preset volume and delaying the opening of the exhalation valve until all airflow in the lungs has ceased. Once volume delivery from the ventilator has stopped, airway pressure drops from its peak value to the plateau value as gas is redistributed within the lung.

Power, Ventilator ($\dot{W}$)

The rate of work performed by the ventilator on the patient:

$$\dot{W} = 0.098 \times Paw \times \dot{V}$$

where

$\dot{W}$ = instantaneous ventilator power (watts)

Paw = airway pressure (cm H_2O)

$\dot{V}$ = flow (L/s)

Note: The constant 0.098 is used to convert cm $H_2O \cdot$ L/s to watts.

Pressure Drop

The difference in pressure between a point of higher pressure and another of lower pressure.

Pressure Hold

One type of proximal airway pressure pattern produced by a positive pressure ventilator. It is characterized by a rise in inspiratory pressure to some peak value that is deliberately sustained for the duration of the inspiratory time.

Resistance (Flow Resistance)

A system property that relates the pressure drop causing flow through the system. For a viscous gas flowing through a tube, resistance arises from the interaction among gas molecules and between gas molecules and the tube wall. Resistance can be calculated as the change in pressure difference producing flow divided by the change in flow, where changes in pressure and flow are measured between points in time of equal lung volume:

$$R = \frac{\Delta(P_1 - P_2)}{\Delta \dot{V}} \qquad (5\text{--}5)$$

where

$$R = \text{resistance (cm } H_2O/L/s)$$

$$\Delta(P_1 - P_2) = \text{change in pressure difference across the system from some point 1 to another point 2 (cm } H_2O)$$

$$\Delta \dot{V} = \text{change in flow (L/s)}$$

The system for which resistance is calculated is defined by the points between which the pressure difference is measured. For example, airway resistance (Raw) is a measure of the flow resistance between the airway opening and the alveoli. If measurements of flow and pressure are made at points of equal lung volume (so that pressure changes due to elastic recoil are canceled out), airway resistance can be estimated by the equation

$$Raw = \frac{\Delta(P_{AO} - P_A)}{\Delta \dot{V}} \qquad (5\text{--}6)$$

where

$$Raw = \text{airway resistance (cm } H_2O/L/s)$$

$$P_{AO} = \text{proximal airway pressure (cm } H_2O)$$

$\dot{V}$ = change in flow (L/s)

P_A = alveolar pressure (cm H_2O)

Also

$$R_L = \frac{\Delta(P_{AO} - P_{PL})}{\Delta \dot{V}} \qquad (5\text{--}7)$$

where

R_L = lung resistance (cm $H_2O/L/s$)

$\Delta \dot{V}$ = change in flow (L/s)

P_{PL} = intrapleural pressure (cm H_2O)

Another example is total respiratory resistance, which includes Raw and other resistances due to pulmonary and chest wall tissue motions. The required pressure difference is between the airway opening and the body surface. During mechanical ventilation with a constant flow generator, the change in this pressure difference can be estimated as peak inspiratory pressure minus plateau pressure. Therefore,

$$R_{RS} = \frac{PIP - P_{PLT}}{\dot{V}_I} \qquad (5\text{--}8)$$

where

R_{RS} = respiratory system resistance (cm $H_2O/L/s$)

PIP = peak inspiratory pressure (cm H_2O)

P_{PLT} = plateau pressure (cm H_2O)

$\dot{V}_I$ = set inspiratory flow rate (L/s)

The major component of R_{RS} and R_L is Raw. Therefore, in practice, they are often used interchangeably as close estimates of each other.

Sigh, Ventilator

A deliberate increase in tidal volume for one or more breaths at intervals. During mechanical ventilation, the sigh volume generally used is twice the tidal volume. During normal spontaneous breathing, sighs occur 6–10 times per hour.

Specific Compliance (C/VL)

A parameter used to characterize the elastic behavior of the material from which a system is made. This is in contrast to compliance, C, which characterizes the elastic behavior of a particular system constructed from the material. Specific compliance is defined as C divided by the total volume of the structure at which C is evaluated. Specific compliance provides a means of comparing the elastic behavior of the pulmonary parenchyma of lungs of different sizes.

Tidal Volume (VT)

The volume change of the patient's lungs during spontaneous breathing or mechanical ventilation. For volume-limited ventilation, the tidal volume is controlled by ventilator settings and remains relatively constant while the pressure necessary to deliver the volume varies with changing lung mechanics. The tidal volume delivered to the patient is usually less than the volume set on the ventilator due to the volume lost (compressed) in the patient system:

$$\text{tidal volume} = \text{set machine volume} - \text{compressed volume}$$

The compressed volume can be calculated if the compliance of the patient circuit (CPC) is known (see Compliance). Once the patient is connected to the ventilator, the compressed volume is determined by the change in airway pressure during inspiration. For example,

$$\text{compressed volume} = (\text{PIP} - \text{PEEP}) \times \text{CPC}$$

where

$$\text{PIP} = \text{peak inspiratory pressure} \quad \text{PEEP} = \text{end-expiratory pressure}$$

During mechanical ventilation, respiratory system compliance affects the change in airway pressure and hence the volume of gas compressed in the patient circuit. If an inspiratory hold maneuver is used, the following equation applies:

$$\text{tidal volume} = \left(\frac{1}{1 + \dfrac{\text{CPC}}{\text{CRS}}} \right) \times \text{set machine volume}$$

where

$$\text{CRS} = \text{respiratory system compliance}$$

If an inspiratory hold is not used, substitute the patient's dynamic characteristic for CRS in this equation.

During pressure control ventilation, the proximal airway pressure pattern is controlled by ventilator settings and remains relatively constant while the tidal volume varies with changing lung mechanics. The change in lung volume caused by a step change in airway pressure (rectangular pressure pattern) is given by

$$V(t) = C \times \Delta P \times (1 - e^{-t/(R \times C)}) = C\Delta P\left(1 - \frac{1}{e^{t/(R \times C)}}\right)$$

where

$V(t)$ = lung volume (L) as a function of time (t). If time = inspiratory time then $V(t)$ = tidal volume.

C = total respiratory system compliance (L/cm H_2O)

ΔP = step change in airway pressure, or PIP − PEEP (cm H_2O)

e = the base of the natural logarithms (approximately 2.72)

t = the time interval (in seconds) from the initiation of the step change in airway pressure; inspiratory time

R = total respiratory system resistance (cm $H_2O/L/s$)

Note: This equation is derived from the equation describing the change in alveolar pressure in response to a step change in airway pressure (see Time Constant).

Time Constant (Resistance × Compliance)

A measure of the time (usually seconds) necessary for an exponential function of time to attain 63% of its value at time equal to infinity. For example, in physiology the respiratory system is often modeled as being composed of a single compliance (representing the chest wall and the alveoli) and a single resistance (representing the airways). If a step input (instantaneous change) of pressure is applied to the airway opening of such a model, the pressure rise in the compliant chamber will be an exponential function of time. To illustrate this, consider the relation governing the mechanics of a completely passive total respiratory system (i.e., one in which all the respiratory muscles are completely relaxed or paralyzed):

$$P_{TR} = \frac{V}{C} + R \times \dot{V} \qquad (5\text{--}9)$$

in which P_{TR} is transrespiratory system pressure, that is, the difference between the pressure at the airway opening and the pressure on the body surface (usually atmospheric pressure). This equation states that the pressure necessary for inflation or deflation of the lungs depends on the compliance of the total respiratory system (C), tidal volume volume (V), resistance (R), and gas flow rate into the lungs ($\dot{V}_L$). For a step change in airway pressure (e.g., $\Delta P_{AO} = PIP - PEEP$), equation (5–9) can be solved for alveolar (lung) pressure as a function of time, assuming resistance and compliance are constant:

$$P_A(t) = \Delta P_{AO} \times (1 - e^{-t/(R \times C)}) \qquad (5\text{–}10)$$

where

$P_A(t)$ = alveolar pressure as a function of time (t)

ΔP_{AO} = change in pressure at the airway opening

e = the base of the natural logarithms (approximately 2.72)

t = the time interval (in seconds) from the initiation of the step change in airway pressure; inspiratory time

This states that the alveolar pressure (the pressure in the compliant chamber in our model) will undergo an exponential change in response to a step change of ΔP in airway pressure. If both sides of equation (5–10) are multiplied by C, we get the equation for lung volume as a function of time (see Tidal Volume).

The product of resistance and compliance, RC (which has the dimensions of time), appears as a fundamental quantity in this equation and is therefore given its own name, the time constant. To appreciate the properties of the time constant, consider the values equation (5–10) will have at specific instants of time. When t is equal to $R \times C$, the term t/RC equals 1 and the expression $1 - e^{-t/R \times C} = 1 - 2.72^{-1} = 1 - 0.37 = 0.63$. Thus, the alveolar pressure is equal to 63% of the forcing pressure, ΔP, when t equals RC. If t is equal to 2RC or two time constants, the alveolar pressure will be 86.5% of the forcing pressure. Alveolar pressure is generally considered to be at its steady-state value when t is equal to 5RC. At this time also, P_A is considered in equilibrium with the pressure at the airway opening, since all flow through the airways has essentially ceased. Expressing t as a multiple of the time constant is thus a convenient method of predicting the time necessary for the system to respond to a step input of pressure. Conversely, the time necessary to attain 63% of the final response (which may be measured experimentally) is equal to the product of R and C and thus gives a mechanical characteristic of the system. Figure 5–4 shows the fraction of ΔP that exists in the lungs at the end of time constants 0 through 5.

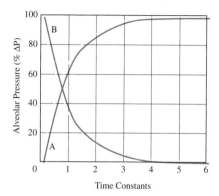

Figure 5-4 Time constant curves. Curve A corresponds to the inspiratory lung pressure and volume and expiratory flow. Curve B corresponds to expiratory lung pressure and volume and inspiratory flow.

Torr

Unit of pressure named in honor of Evangelista Torricelli, who invented the mercury barometer. The torr is defined as exactly equal to 1/760 of a standard atmosphere. It is generally considered to be equal to a millimeter of mercury, although the latter is gravity-dependent.

Total Cycle Time (TCT)

The time necessary for one complete respiratory cycle.

$$TCT = T_I + T_E = \frac{60}{f}$$

where

$$TCT = \text{total cycle time (s)}$$
$$T_I = \text{inspiratory time (s)}$$
$$T_E = \text{expiratory time (s)}$$
$$f = \text{ventilatory frequency (breaths/min)}$$

Trigger

To trigger the ventilator means to initiate the inspiratory time.

Work, Ventilator (W)

Work performed by the ventilator on the patient:

$$W = 0.098 \times \int P \times \dot{V}\, dt$$

where

   W = work (joules)

   P = pressure (cm H_2O)

   $\dot{V}$ = flow (L/s)

   0.098 = constant to convert cm $H_2O \cdot L$ to joules

■ CLASSIFYING MODES OF MECHANICAL VENTILATION

A "mode" of mechanical ventilation can be generally defined as a predetermined pattern of interaction between a ventilator and a patient. There are over 100 names for modes of ventilation on commercially available mechanical ventilators. Neither the manufacturing community nor the medical community has developed a standard taxonomy for modes. However, we present here an approach to both defining and classifying the major characteristics of modes. It consists of 10 fundamental aphorisms that constitute the components of a practical taxonomy and ultimately, an adequately explicit definition of "mode." The aphorisms are given in outline form below:

1. **The Breath.** The normal breathing pattern is cyclic and thus a breath is conveniently characterized by the phases of the flow–time waveform at the airway opening.

   1.1. The positive phase of the flow waveform is designated inspiration (inspiratory phase). The negative phase of the flow waveform and the remaining time until the next inspiration indicates expiration (expiratory phase).

      1.1.1. Inspiration (inspiratory time) includes the phase of positive flow and any period of zero flow before flow goes negative.

      1.1.2. Expiration (expiratory time) includes the phase of negative flow and any period of zero flow before flow goes positive for the next cycle.

2. **The Assisted Breath.** A ventilator can provide all of the mechanical work of inspiration or only a portion of it.

    2.1. An assisted breath is one for which the ventilator does some or all of the work of breathing (i.e., transrespiratory pressure rises during inspiration or falls during expiration).

    2.2. An unassisted breath is one for which the ventilator simply provides flow at the rate required by the patient's inspiratory effort (i.e., transrespiratory system pressure stays constant throughout the breath).

    2.3. A loaded breath is one for which the patient does work on the ventilator (i.e., transrespiratory pressure falls during inspiration or rises during expiration).

3. **The Control Variable.** Ventilators operate by manipulating a control variable. For simple control systems, where pressure, volume, or flow is preset, the control variable is the independent variable in the equation of motion for the respiratory system. In more complicated schemes, the control variable is identified according to the feedback loop that is predominant within a breath (not between breaths). For example, with Proportional Assist, pressure, volume, and flow all vary during the breath, and none of them are preset. However, the targeting scheme is designed to control pressure such that it satisfies the equation of motion for preset values of respiratory system elastance and resistance that are to be supported for any instantaneous values of inspiratory flow and volume generated by the patient's inspiratory effort.

    3.1. For historical reasons and to simplify descriptions of ventilator operation, pressure and volume are considered to be the control variables.

        3.1.1. Volume is measured and controlled either directly (e.g., by the excursion of a piston) or indirectly (by integration of the flow signal).

    3.2. While a ventilator can control only one variable, it may switch from volume control to pressure control or vice versa during an individual inspiration.

4. **Trigger and Cycle Variables.** During mechanical ventilation, an individual breath is classified by the criteria that start (trigger) and end (cycle) the inspiratory phase.

   4.1. Inspiratory time is determined by the cycle criterion.

   4.2. Expiratory time is determined by the trigger criterion.

   4.3. The duration of the breath (total cycle time) is the sum of the inspiratory and expiratory times.

   4.4. These criteria may be set either as static values for each breath (e.g., operator preset) or as dynamic values determined by algorithms during the course of ventilation.

5. **Patient and Machine Triggering and Cycling.** Trigger and cycle criteria can be grouped into two categories: machine initiated and patient initiated.

   5.1. Machine-initiated criteria are those that determine the start and end of the inspiratory phase independent of the patient. This means that the ventilator determines the inspiratory time and expiratory time, or alternatively, the inspiratory time and frequency.

      5.1.1. **Machine triggering** criteria include but are not limited to:

         5.1.1.1. Frequency

         5.1.1.2. Expiratory time

         5.1.1.3. Minimum minute ventilation

      5.1.2. **Machine cycling** criteria include:

         5.1.2.1. Inspiratory time

         5.1.2.2. Tidal volume

   5.2. Patient-initiated criteria are those that affect the start and end of the inspiratory phase independent of any machine settings for inspiratory and expiratory time. This means that the patient may affect the inspiratory time and frequency.

      5.2.1. **Patient triggering** criteria include but are not limited to:

         5.2.1.1. Transrespiratory system pressure

         5.2.1.2. Inspiratory volume

         5.2.1.3. Inspiratory flow

        5.2.1.4. Diaphragmatic electromyogram

        5.2.1.5. Transthoracic electrical impedance

    5.2.2. **Patient cycling** criteria include:

        5.2.2.1. Transrespiratory system pressure

        5.2.2.2. Inspiratory flow

6. **Mandatory and Spontaneous Breaths.** An individual breath is classified as being mandatory or spontaneous. A mandatory breath is one for which the start or end of inspiration (or both) is determined by the ventilator, according to a preset schedule (e.g., preset frequency or minute ventilation). Mandatory breaths will begin and end without a signal from the patient but may also be synchronized with a patient signal (e.g., change in baseline pressure or flow). A spontaneous breath is one for which the start and end of inspiration is determined by the patient. Triggering and cycling of a spontaneous breath may occur due to a signal derived from active inspiratory or expiratory efforts or a signal derived from the passive behavior of the respiratory system (e.g., change in pressure or flow during inspiration or expiration governed by the time constant of the respiratory system).

    6.1. Mandatory breaths are machine triggered or machine cycled or both.

    6.2. Spontaneous breaths are both patient triggered and patient cycled.

7. **The Breath Sequence.** A breath sequence is a particular pattern of mandatory and/or spontaneous breaths. Breath sequences can be grouped into three categories:

    7.1. **Continuous mandatory ventilation (CMV):** Mandatory breaths are patient triggered for every patient effort that satisfies the mandatory breath trigger criteria. In the absence of patient triggering, mandatory breaths will be machine triggered. Spontaneous breaths may occur during a mandatory inspiration but not between mandatory breaths.

    7.2. **Intermittent mandatory ventilation (IMV):** Mandatory breaths are patient triggered if the patient effort satisfies the mandatory breath trigger criteria and it occurs in a brief trigger window, which typically occurs at the end of the expiratory time allowed by the preset mandatory breath frequency. Otherwise they are machine triggered, and spontaneous breaths may occur between mandatory breaths.

7.2.1. If the frequency of either spontaneous breaths or patient-triggered mandatory breaths is too low, mandatory breaths may be machine triggered. Three common variations of IMV are:

7.2.1.1. Mandatory breaths are always delivered at the set frequency.

7.2.1.2. Mandatory breaths are delivered only when the spontaneous breath frequency falls below the set frequency.

7.2.1.3. Mandatory breaths are delivered only when the spontaneous minute ventilation (i.e., product of spontaneous breath frequency and spontaneous breath tidal volume) drops below a preset or computed threshold (also known as mandatory minute ventilation).

7.2.2. Spontaneous breaths may occur during a mandatory inspiration.

7.3. **Continuous spontaneous ventilation (CSV):** Every breath is spontaneous.

8. **The Ventilatory Pattern.** A ventilatory pattern is a specification for a particular control variable associated with a particular breath sequence. There are five basic ventilatory patterns:

8.1. Volume-controlled continuous mandatory ventilation (VC-CMV)

8.2. Volume-controlled intermittent mandatory ventilation (VC-IMV)

8.3. Pressure-controlled continuous mandatory ventilation (PC-CMV)

8.4. Pressure-controlled intermittent mandatory ventilation (PC-IMV)

8.5. Pressure-controlled continuous spontaneous ventilation (PC-CSV)

8.5.1. All forms of CSV are either uncontrolled (i.e., the ventilator does nothing) or forms of pressure control. Therefore PC-CSV may be abbreviated as CSV.

9. **Targeting Schemes.** During inspiration, the control variable can be manipulated by a variety of feedback control or targeting schemes. These schemes can be ranked according to complexity and degree

of required operator intervention. Common examples include the following:

9.1. **Setpoint control:** the operator is required to preset all parameters of the breath (i.e., pressure, volume, flow, and timing)

9.2. **Dual control:** the operator presets pressure, volume, flow, and timing parameters and the ventilator switches between volume control and pressure control, within a single breath, based on the preset parameters.

9.3. **Servo control:** the ventilator delivers pressure in proportion to the patient-generated volume and/or flow according to a preset model (e.g., the equation of motion). Model parameters are preset by the operator.

9.4. **Adaptive control:** the ventilator automatically adjusts one or more breath setpoints based on other operator preset criteria (e.g., the ventilator adjusts peak inspiratory pressure to achieve an average preset target tidal volume).

9.5. **Optimum control:** the ventilator automatically adjusts one or more setpoints based a model that attempts to minimize or maximize some other variable(s). Parameters of the model may be preset by the operator.

9.6. **Intelligent control:** the ventilator automatically adjusts one or more setpoints based on an artificial intelligence program.

10. **Modes of Ventilation.** The control variable (i.e., volume or pressure), the ventilatory pattern, and the targeting scheme are the levels of a taxonomy for modes of ventilation analogous to the family, genus, and species taxonomy for animals. For example, BiPAP and Adaptive Support Ventilation are different modes of the PC-IMV ventilatory pattern in the pressure control family just as lions and tigers are different species in the genus panther in the family of cats. A mode of ventilation, therefore, is a complete specification for preset ventilator-patient interaction. A mode description comprises a unique combination of control variable, ventilatory pattern, targeting scheme, and other relevant operational algorithms. A mode may also be referred to by a name, such as "pressure support" or "SmartCare."

10.1. Any mode of ventilation can be associated with one and only one ventilatory pattern.

10.2. Modes within a particular ventilatory pattern are distinguished by their targeting scheme, the trigger and cycle criteria, and any other unique operational algorithm feature. The finer the distinction required, the more levels of criteria that are needed.

Table 5-10 shows how this system can be used to classify a variety of modes of ventilation.

Table 5-10 A selection of modes named by manufacturers classified using the taxonomy built from the 10 aphorisms

Control Variable	Breath Sequence	Targeting Scheme	Example Modes
Volume Control	CMV	SetPoint	Volume Control, VC-A/C, CMV, (S)CMV, Assist/Control
		Dual	CMV + Pressure Limited
		Adaptive	Adaptive Flow
	IMV	SetPoint	SIMV, VC-SIMV
		Dual	SIMV + Pressure Limited
		Adaptive	AutoMode (VC-VS), Mandatory Minute Volume
Pressure Control	CMV	SetPoint	Pressure Control, PC-A/C, AC PCV, HFO, HFJV
		Adaptive	Pressure Regulated Volume Control, VC+A/C, CMV+AutoFlow
	IMV	SetPoint	Airway Pressure Release Ventilation SIMV PCV, BiLevel, PiPAP S/T, DuoPAP, PCV+
		Adaptive	VC + SIMV, V V + SIMV, SIMV + AutoFlow, Automode (PRVC-VS)
		Optimal	Adaptive Support Ventilation
Pressure Control	CSV	SetPoint	CPAP, Pressure Support
		Dual	Volume Assured Pressure Support
		Servo	Proportional Assist Ventilation, Automatic Tube Compensation
		Adaptive	Volume Support
		Intelligent	SmartCare, Adaptive Support Ventilation

VC = volume control; PC = pressure control; CMV = continuous mandatory ventilation; IMV = intermittent mandatory ventilation; CSV = continuous spontaneous ventilation.

■ MATHEMATICAL MODELS OF PRESSURE-CONTROLLED MECHANICAL VENTILATION

Reference: *J Appl Physiol* 67(3) (1982), 1081–1092.

Glossary

C	compliance (L/cm H_2O)
D	inspiratory time fraction (T_I/T_{TOT})
f	frequency (breaths/min)
R_E	expiratory resistance (cm $H_2O \cdot L^{-1} \cdot s$)
R_I	inspiratory resistance (cm $H_2O \cdot L^{-1} \cdot s$)
T_E	expiratory time (s)
T_I	inspiratory time (s)
TCT	total cycle time (s) = $T_I + T_E$ = f/60
$\dot{V}_E$	minute ventilation (L/min)
V_T	tidal volume
W	inspiratory work per breath (J)
$\dot{W}$	power of breathing; rate of work (J/min)
τ_I	inspiratory time constant (s) = $C \cdot R_I$
τ_E	expiratory time constant (s) = $C \cdot R_E$
PIP	peak inspiratory pressure above set PEEP (cm H_2O)
P_A	alveolar pressure above set PEEP (cm H_2O)
$\overline{P}_{AW}$	mean airway pressure above set PEEP (cm H_2O)
$\overline{P}_A$	mean alveolar pressure above set PEEP (cm H_2O)
P_{SET}	preset constant inspiratory pressure above preset PEEP during pressure controlled ventilation (cm H_2O)
PEEP	preset positive end-expiratory airway pressure
P_{EE}	end-expiratory alveolar pressure or autoPEEP (cm H_2O)

Model Assumptions

1. The pressure applied at the airway opening represents the entire pressure difference acting on the respiratory system; passive conditions exist throughout the ventilatory cycle.

2. The pressure applied to the airway opening rises immediately to P_{SET} during inspiration and falls immediately to PEEP during expiration; a rectangular pressure–time waveform is assumed.

3. The units for each variable are those commonly used clinically:

   a. Time (seconds, s)

   b. Pressure (cm H_2O)

   c. Volume (liters, L)

   d. Resistance (cm $H_2O \cdot s \cdot L^{-1}$)

   e. Compliance (L/cm H_2O)

   f. Frequency (breaths/min)

For inspiration, assuming $P_{EE} = 0$

$$V(t) = C \cdot P_{SET}(1 - e^{-t/\tau_I})$$

$$P_A(t) = P_{SET}(1 - e^{-t/\tau_I}) + PEEP$$

$$\dot{V}_I(t) = \left(\frac{P_{SET}}{R_I}\right)e^{-t/\tau_I}$$

For single expiration, assuming $P_{EE} = 0$

$$V(t) = C \cdot P_{SET}(e^{-t/\tau_E})$$

$$P_A(t) = P_{SET}(e^{-t/\tau_E}) + PEEP$$

$$\dot{V}_I(t) = -\left(\frac{P_{SET}}{R_I}\right)e^{-t/\tau_E}$$

General equations, assuming $P_{EE} \neq 0$

$$V_T = \frac{(P_{SET} \cdot C)(1 - e^{-T_I/\tau_I})(1 - e^{-T_E/\tau_E})}{(1 - e^{-T_I/\tau_I} \cdot e^{-T_E/\tau_E})}$$

$$V_T = \frac{(P_{SET} \cdot C)(1 - e^{-60D/fR_IC})[1 - e^{-60(1-D)/fR_EC}]}{(1 - e^{-60D/fR_IC} \cdot e^{-60(1-D)/fR_EC})}$$

$$P_{EE} = \frac{\dot{V}_E(e^{-T_E/\tau_E})}{f \cdot C(1 - e^{-T_E/\tau_E})} + PEEP = \frac{V_T(e^{-T_E/\tau_E})}{C(1 - e^{-T_E/\tau_E})} + PEEP$$

$$P_{EE} = \frac{P_{SET}(e^{-T_E/\tau_E})(1 - e^{-T_I/\tau_I})}{(1 - e^{-T_I/\tau_I} \cdot e^{-T_E/\tau_E})} + PEEP$$

$$\text{P}_{\text{EE}} = \frac{\dot{\text{V}}_{\text{E}}\left[e^{-\,60(1-\text{D})/f\text{REC}}\right]}{f \cdot C\left[1 - e^{-60(1-\text{D})/f\text{REC}}\right]} + \text{PEEP} = \frac{\text{V}_{\text{T}}\left[e^{-60(1-\text{D})/f\text{REC}}\right]}{C\left[1 - e^{-60(1-\text{D})f\text{REC}}\right]} + \text{PEEP}$$

$$\overline{\text{P}}_{\text{A}} = \{(\text{TCT}/C) \cdot [(\text{P}_{\text{SET}} \cdot C \cdot \text{T}_{\text{I}}) - (\text{P}_{\text{SET}} \cdot C - \text{V}_{\text{EE}})(\tau_{\text{I}})(1 - e^{-\text{T}_{\text{I}}/\tau_{\text{I}}})$$

$$+ (\text{V}_{\text{T}} + \text{V}_{\text{EE}})(\tau_{\text{E}})(1 - e^{-\text{T}_{\text{E}}/\tau_{\text{E}}})]\} + \text{PEEP}$$

where

$$\text{V}_{\text{EE}} = \frac{\text{V}_{\text{T}}(e^{-\text{T}_{\text{E}}/\tau_{\text{E}}})}{1 - e^{-\text{T}_{\text{E}}/\tau_{\text{E}}}}$$

$$\text{P}_{\text{A}} = \left[\frac{\text{P}_{\text{SET}}(1 - e^{\text{T}_{\text{I}}/\tau_{\text{I}}})}{1 - e^{-\text{T}_{\text{I}}/\tau_{\text{I}}} \cdot e^{-\text{T}_{\text{E}}/\tau_{\text{E}}}}\right] + \text{PEEP}$$

$$\text{W} = C \cdot \text{P}_{\text{SET}}(\text{P}_{\text{SET}} - \text{P}_{\text{EE}})(1 - e^{\text{T}_{\text{I}}/\tau_{\text{I}}})$$

$$\dot{\text{W}} = f \cdot C \cdot \text{P}_{\text{SET}}(\text{P}_{\text{SET}} - \text{P}_{\text{EE}})(1 - e^{\text{T}_{\text{I}}/\tau_{\text{I}}})$$

6

Mathematical Procedures

The multidisciplinary approach to medicine has incorporated a wide variety of mathematical procedures from the fields of physics, chemistry, and engineering. The information presented in this chapter is designed as a self-teaching refresher course to be used as a review of basic mathematical procedures. Some of the more advanced mathematical concepts, including the section on descriptive statistics, should also help the practitioner to interpret data presented in medical journals and scientific articles.

■ FUNDAMENTAL AXIOMS

Commutative Axiom

$$a + b = b + a$$

$$ab = ba$$

When two or more numbers are added or multiplied together, their order does not affect the result.

Associative Axiom

$$(a + b) + c = a + (b + c)$$

$$(ab)c = a(bc)$$

When three or more numbers are added together, the way they are grouped or associated makes no difference in the result. The same holds true for multiplication.

Distributive Axiom

$$a(b + c) = ab + ac$$

A coefficient (multiplier) of a sum may be distributed as a multiplier of each term.

Order of Precedence

A convention has been established for the order in which numerical operations are performed. This is to prevent confusion when evaluating expressions such as 2×3^2, which could be either 18 or 36. The following rules apply:

1. If the numerical expression *does not* contain fences (such as parentheses), then operations are carried out in the following order:

   a. Raising numbers to powers or extracting roots of numbers.

   b. Multiplication or division.

   c. Addition or subtraction.

Example

$$4 \times 5 + 8 \div 2 + 6^2 - \sqrt{16} + 1 = 20 + 4 + 36 - 4 + 1 = 57$$

2. If the numerical expression *does* contain fences, then follow the procedure in Rule 1, starting with the *innermost* set of parentheses. The sequence is round fences (parentheses), square fences [brackets], double fences {braces}. Once the fences have been eliminated, the expression can be evaluated following Rule 1.

Example

$$2 + 4 \times \{3 \times 2 - [5 \times 4 + (2 \times 3 - 4 \div 1) - 20] + 12\}$$
$$= 2 + 4 \times \{3 \times 2 - [5 \times 4 + (6 - 4) - 20] + 12\}$$
$$= 2 + 4 \times \{3 \times 2 - [5 \times 4 + 2 - 20] + 12\}$$
$$= 2 + 4 \times \{3 \times 2 - [20 + 2 - 20] + 12\}$$
$$= 2 + 4 \times \{3 \times 2 - 2 + 12\}$$
$$= 2 + 4 \times \{6 - 2 + 12\}$$
$$= 2 + 4 \times 16$$
$$2 + 64 = 66$$

■ FRACTIONS

When a number is expressed as a fraction (e.g., $\frac{3}{5}$), the number above the line (3) is called the **numerator** and the number below the line (5) the **denominator**.

Multiplication Property of Fractions

$$\frac{a \times c}{b \times c} = \frac{a}{b} \qquad (c \neq 0)$$

The numerator and denominator of a fraction may be multiplied or divided by the same nonzero number to produce a fraction of equal value.

Example
Simplify (reduce) the fraction $\dfrac{9}{12}$

Solution	
1. Find the largest integer that will evenly divide both the numerator and denominator.	The largest whole number is 3.
2. Divide both the numerator and denominator by that number.	$\dfrac{9}{12} = \left(\dfrac{9}{3}\right) \div \left(\dfrac{12}{3}\right) = \dfrac{3}{4}$

Multiplication of Fractions

$$\frac{a}{b} \times \frac{c}{d} = \frac{ac}{bd}$$

Example
$\dfrac{7}{9} \times \dfrac{3}{4} = ?$

Solution	
1. Multiply the numerators.	$7 \times 3 = 21$
2. Multiply the denominators.	$9 \times 4 = 36$
3. Simplify the resulting fraction if possible.	$\dfrac{7}{9} \times \dfrac{3}{4} = \dfrac{21}{36}$
	$= \dfrac{7}{12}$

Division of Fractions

$$\frac{a}{b} \div \frac{c}{d} = \frac{a}{b} \times \frac{d}{c} = \frac{ad}{bc}$$

Example	
	Find the quotient: $\dfrac{5}{8} \div \dfrac{2}{3}$

Solution	
1. Invert the divisor.	Change $\dfrac{2}{3}$ to $\dfrac{3}{2}$
2. Multiply the dividend by the inverted divisor.	$\dfrac{5}{8} \times \dfrac{3}{2} = \dfrac{15}{16}$
3. Simplify if possible.	

Addition and Subtraction of Fractions with the Same Denominator

$$\frac{a}{b} + \frac{c}{b} = \frac{(a + c)}{b}$$

$$\frac{a}{b} - \frac{c}{b} = \frac{(a - c)}{b}$$

Example	
	$\dfrac{5}{32} + \dfrac{13}{32} - \dfrac{3}{32} = ?$

Solution	
1. Combine numerators.	$5 + 13 - 3 = 15$
2. Write the resultant fraction with the new numerator and the same denominator.	$\dfrac{15}{32}$
3. Simplify if possible.	

Addition and Subtraction of Fractions with Different Denominators

To add or subtract fractions that do not have the same denominator, it is first necessary to express them as fractions having the same denominators. To find a common denominator, find an integer that is evenly divisible by each denominator. The smallest or least common denominator (LCD) is the most convenient.

Example
$$\frac{5}{4} + \frac{7}{18} = ?$$

Solution

1. First find the LCD as follows:

   a. Express each denominator as the product of primes (integers greater than 1 that are evenly divisible by only themselves and 1).

   a. $4 = 2 \times 2 = 2^2$
   $18 = 2 \times 3 \times 3$
   $= 2 \times 3^2$

   b. Note the greatest power to which an integer occurs in any denominator.

   b. 2^2 is the greatest power of 2 in either denominator, 3^2 is the greatest power of 3 in either denominator.

   c. The product of the integers noted in part b is the LCD.

   c. $2^2 \times 3^2 = 36$

2. Write fractions as equivalent fractions with denominators equal to the LCD.

   $$\frac{5}{4} \times \frac{9}{9} = \frac{45}{36}$$

   $$\frac{7}{18} \times \frac{2}{2} = \frac{14}{36}$$

3. Combine the numerators and use the LCD as the denominator.

   $$\frac{45}{36} + \frac{14}{36} = \frac{59}{36}$$
   $$= 1.64$$

4. Simplify if possible.

■ RATIOS, PROPORTIONS, AND UNIT CONVERSION

The **ratio** of two numbers may be written as follows:

$$a/b = a:b$$

Two equivalent ratios form a **proportion**.

$$a/b = c/d$$

$$a:b = c:d$$

$$a:b :: c:d$$

Regardless of how the above proportions are expressed, they are read "*a* is to *b* as *c* is to *d*."

Ratios provide a convenient method for converting units. To change the units of a quantity, multiply by ratios whose values are equal to 1 (which does not change the value of the quantity). Select the dimensions of the ratios such that the unit to be changed occurs as a factor of the numerator or as a factor of the denominator. Thus, when the quantity is multiplied by the ratio, the unit is canceled and replaced by an equivalent unit and quantity.

Example
Convert 2 kilometers/hour to feet/second.

Solution	
1. Write an equation expressing the problem.	2 km/hr = x ft/s
2. Multiply the known quantity by ratios whose value is equal to 1, such that the desired unit remains after canceling pairs of equal dimensions that appear in both the numerator and the denominator.	1 km = 1,000 m 1 m = 3.281 ft 1 hr = 60 min 1 min = 60 s

$$\frac{2\ \text{km}}{\text{hr}} \times \frac{1,000\ \text{m}}{1\ \text{km}} \times \frac{3.3\ \text{ft}}{1\ \text{m}} \times \frac{1\ \text{hr}}{60\ \text{min}} \times \frac{1\ \text{min}}{60\ \text{s}} = \frac{6,600\ \text{ft}}{3,600\ \text{s}} = \frac{1.8\ \text{ft}}{\text{s}}$$

■ EXPONENTS

When a product is the result of multiplying a factor by itself several times, it is convenient to use a shorthand notation that shows the number used as a factor (a) and the number of factors (n) in the product. In general, such numbers are expressed in the form a^n, where a is the **base** and n the **exponent**. The rules for these numbers are shown in Table 6–7.

Table 6-7 Rules for Exponents

Rule	Example
$a^n \cdot a^m = a^{n+m}$	$x^2 \cdot x^3 = x^5$
$a^n \div a^m = a^{n-m}$	$z^7 \div z^5 = z^2$
$(ab)^n = a^n b^n$	$(2wy)^2 = 4w^2 y^2$
$a^0 = 1, (a \neq 0)$	$9x^0 = 9$
$a^1 = a$	$3x^1 = 3x$
$a^{-n} = 1/a^n$	$x^{-2} = 1/x^2$
$a^{1/n} = \sqrt[n]{a}$	$y^{1/3} = \sqrt[3]{y}$
$a^{m/n} = \sqrt[n]{a^m}$	$z^{2/3} = \sqrt[3]{z^2}$
$(a^m)^n = a^{mn}$	$(w^2)^3 = w^6$

■ SCIENTIFIC NOTATION

A number expressed as a multiple of a power of 10, such as 3.02×10^5, is said to be written in **scientific notation**. Numbers written in this way have two parts: a number between 1 and 10 called the **coefficient**, multiplied by a power of 10 called the **exponent**. This notation has three distinct advantages:

a. It simplifies the expression of very large or very small numbers that would otherwise require many zeros. For example, $681,000,000 = 6.81 \times 10^8$ and $0.000026 = 2.6 \times 10^{-5}$.

b. Scientific notation clarifies the number of significant figures in a large number. For example, if the radius of the earth is written as 6,378,000 m, it is not clear whether any of the zeros after the 8 is significant. However, when the same number is written as 6.378×10^6 m, it is understood that only the first four digits are significant.

c. Calculations that involve very large or very small numbers are greatly simplified using scientific notation.

Addition and Subtraction

Example
$6.18 \times 10^3 + 1.9 \times 10^2 - 5.0 \times 10^1$

Solution	
1. Convert all numbers to the same power of 10 as the number with the highest exponent.	$6.18 \times 10^3 = 6.18 \times 10^3$ $1.9 \times 10^2 = 0.19 \times 10^3$ $5.0 \times 10^1 = 0.05 \times 10^3$
2. Add or subtract the coefficients and retain the same exponent in the answer.	6.18×10^3 $+ \ 0.19 \times 10^3$ $- \ 0.05 \times 10^3$ $\overline{6.32 \times 10^3}$

Multiplication and Division

Example
$(4 \times 10^{23})(2 \times 10^{14})$

Solution	
1. Multiply (or divide) the coefficients.	$(4 \times 10^{23})(2 \times 10^{14})$ $= 8(10^{23} \times 10^{14})$
2. Combine the powers of 10 using the rules for exponents.	$8(10^{23} \times 10^{14})$ $= 8 \times 10^{23 + 14}$ $= 8 \times 10^{37}$

Powers and Roots

Example
$(4 \times 10^5)^2$

Solution	
1. Raise the coefficient to the indicated power.	$(4 \times 10^5)^2 = (4^2)(10^5)^2$ $= 16(10^5)^2$
2. Multiply the exponent by the indicated power.	$16(10^5)^2 = 16(10^{5 \times 2})$ $= 16 \times 10^{10}$ $= 1.6 \times 10^{11}$

■ SIGNIFICANT FIGURES

By convention, the number of digits used to express a measured number roughly indicates the error. For example, if a measurement is reported as 35.2 cm, one would assume that the true length was between 35.15 and 35.24 cm (i.e., the error is about 0.05 cm). The last digit (2) in the reported measurement is uncertain, although one can reliably state that it is either 1 or 2. The digit to the right of 2, however, can be any number (5, 6, 7, 8, 9, 0, 1, 2, 3, 4). If the measurement is reported as 35.20 cm, it would indicate that the error is even less (0.005 cm). The number of reliably known digits in a measurement is the number of **significant figures**. Thus, the number 35.2 cm has three significant figures, and the number 35.20 cm has four. The number of significant figures is independent of the decimal point. The numbers 35.2 cm and 0.352 m are the same quantities, both having three significant figures and expressing the same degree of accuracy. The use of significant figures to indicate the accuracy of a result is not as precise as giving the actual error, but is sufficient for most purposes.

Zeros as Significant Figures

Final zeros to the right of the decimal point that are used to indicate accuracy are significant:

179.0   4 significant figures
28.600   5 significant figures
0.30   2 significant figures

For numbers less than one, zeros between the decimal point and the first digit are *not* significant:

0.09   1 significant figure
0.00010   2 significant figures

Zeros between digits are significant:

10.5   3 significant figures
0.8070   4 significant figures
6000.01   6 significant figures

If a number is written with no decimal point, the final zeros may or may not be significant. For instance, the distance between Earth and the sun might be written as 92,900,000 miles, although the accuracy may be only ±5000 miles. This would make only the first zero after the 9 significant. On the other hand, a value of 50 mL measured with a graduated cylinder would be expected to have two significant figures owing to the greater accuracy of the measurement. To avoid ambiguity, numbers are often written as powers of 10 (scientific notation), making all digits significant. Using this convention, 92,900,000 would be written 9.290×10^7, indicating that there are four significant figures.

Calculations Using Significant Figures

The least precise measurement used in a calculation determines the number of significant figures in the answer. Thus, $73.5 + 0.418 = 73.9$ rather than 73.918, since the least precise number (73.5) is accurate to only one decimal place. Similarly, $0.394 - 0.3862 = 0.008$, with only one significant figure.

For multiplication or division, the rule of thumb is: The product or quotient has the same number of significant figures as the term with the fewest significant figures. As an example, in $28.08 \times 4.6/79.4 = 1.6268$, the term with the fewest significant figures is 4.6. Since this number has at most two significant figures, the result should be rounded off to 1.6.

Rounding Off

The results of mathematical computations are often rounded off to specific numbers of significant figures. This is done so that one does not infer an accuracy in the result that was not present in the measurements. The following rules are universally accepted and will ensure bias-free reporting of results (the number of significant figures desired should be determined first).

1. If the final digits of the number are 1, 2, 3, or 4, they are rounded down (dropped) and the preceding figure is retained unaltered.
2. If the final digits are 6, 7, 8, or 9, they are rounded up (i.e., they are dropped and the preceding figure is increased by one).
3. If the digit to be dropped is a 5, it is rounded down if the preceding figure is even and rounded up if the preceding figure is odd. Thus, 2.45 and 6.15 are rounded off to 2.4 and 6.2, respectively.

■ FUNCTIONS

A **function** is a particular type of relation between groups of numbers. The uniqueness of a function is that each member of one group is associated with exactly one member of another group. In general, let the variable x stand for the values of one group of numbers and the variable y stand for the values of another group. If each value of x is associated with a unique value of y, then this relation is a function. Specifically, y is said to be a function of x and is denoted $y = f(x)$. With this notation, x is called the *independent variable* and y the *dependent variable*. A function may be represented graphically by using a two-dimensional coordinate (Cartesian) plane formed by two perpendicular axes intersecting each other at a point with coordinates designated as $x = 0$, $y = 0$ (Fig. 6–1). The vertical axis denotes values of y and the horizontal axis values of x. The function is plotted as a series of points whose coordinates are the values of x with their corresponding values of y as determined by the function.

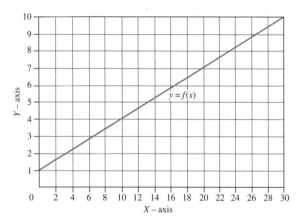

Figure 6-1 Graphic representation of the function y = f(x), where f(x)= 0.3x + 1.

Linear Functions

One of the simplest functions is expressed by the formula

$$y = ax$$

where

> y and x are variables
>
> a is a constant

The constant a is sometimes referred to as the *constant of proportionality* and y is said to be *directly proportional* to x (if y is expressed as $y = a/x$, y is said to be inversely proportional to x and the function is no longer linear). The graph of the equation $y = ax$ is a straight line. The constant a is the *slope* of the line.

General Linear Equation

$$y = ax + b$$

where

> y = dependent variable
>
> a = slope
>
> x = independent variable
>
> b = y-intercept (the value of y at which the graph of the equation crosses the y-axis)

Solving Linear Equations

To solve a linear equation,

1. Combine similar terms.
2. Use inverse operations to undo remaining additions and subtractions (i.e., add or subtract the same quantities to both sides of the equation). Get all terms with the unknown variable on one side of the equation.
3. If the equation involves fractions, multiply both sides by the least common denominator.
4. If there are multiplications or divisions indicated in the variable term, use inverse operations to find the value of the variable.
5. Check the result by substituting the value into the original equation.

Examples

1. $8 + 10x - 40 = 3x + 7 + 2x + \dfrac{2x}{3}$

   $10x - 32 = 5x + \dfrac{2x}{3} + 7$

2. $10x - 32 + 32 = 5x + \dfrac{2x}{3} + 7 + 32$

   $10x = 5x + \dfrac{2x}{3} + 39$

   $10x - 5x - \dfrac{2x}{3} = 39$

   $5x - \dfrac{2x}{3} = 39$

3. $3\left(5x - \dfrac{2x}{3}\right) = 3(39)$

   $15x - 2x = 117$

4. $13x = 117$

   $\dfrac{13x}{13} = \dfrac{117x}{13}$

   $x = 9$

5. $8 + 10(9) - 40 = 3(9) + 7 + 2(9) + \dfrac{2(9)}{3}$

   $8 + 90 - 40 = 27 + 7 + 18 + 6$

   $58 = 58$

■ QUADRATIC EQUATIONS

A function of the form $y = ax^2$ is called a **quadratic function**. It is sometimes expressed in the more general form

$$y = ax^2 + bx + c$$

where

   a, b, and c are constants

The graph of this equation is a *parabola*. Frequently, it is of interest to know where the parabola intersects the x-axis. The value of y at any point on the x-axis is zero. Therefore, to find the values of x where the graph intersects the x-axis, the quadratic equation is expressed in *standard form:*

$$ax^2 + bx + c = 0$$

with $a \neq 0$.

The solution of any quadratic equation expressed in standard form may be found using the **quadratic formula**:

$$x = \frac{-b \pm \sqrt{b^2 - 4ac}}{2a}$$

where

a, b, and c are the coefficients in the quadratic equation

Example
Solve $3x^2 + 7 = 10x$

Solution	
1. Write the equation in standard form.	$3x^2 - 10x + 7 = 0$
2. Note the coefficients a, b, and c.	$a = 3, b = -10, c = 7$
3. Substitute these values in the quadratic formula: $x = \dfrac{-b \pm \sqrt{b^2 - 4ac}}{2a}$	$x = \dfrac{-(-10) \pm \sqrt{(-10)^2 - 4(3)(7)}}{2(3)}$
4. Simplify.	$x = \dfrac{10 \pm \sqrt{100 - 84}}{6}$ $= \dfrac{10 \pm \sqrt{16}}{6}$ $= 2.33 \text{ or } 1$

■ LOGARITHMS

The **logarithm** of a number (N) is the exponent (x) to which the base (a) must be raised to produce N. Thus, if $a^x = N$ then $\log_a N = x$ for $a > 0$ and $a \neq 0$. For example, $\log_2 8 = 3$ (read: the log to the base 2 equals 3) because $2^3 = 8$. Logarithms are written as numbers with two parts: an integer, called the characteristic, and a decimal, called the mantissa (e.g., $\log_{10} 86 = 1.9345$).

Common Logarithms

Common logarithms are those that have the base 10. In this book, the base number will be omitted with the assumption that log means $\log_{10}$. Table 6–1 shows the general rules of common logarithms.

x	log x
$10^0 = 1$	$\log 1 = 0$
$10^1 = 10$	$\log 10 = 1$
$10^2 = 100$	$\log 100 = 2$

Table 6–1 Rules of Common Logarithms

Rule	Example
1. $\log ab = \log a + \log b$ ($a > 0, b > 0$)	$x = (746)(384)$ $\log x = \log 746 + \log 384$ $\log 746 = 2.8727$ $\log 384 = 2.5843$ $\log x = 5.4570$ $x = 286{,}400$
2. $\log 1/a = -\log a$ ($a > 0$)	$x = 1/273$ $\log x = -\log 273$ $= -2.4362$ $= \overline{3}.5638$ $x = 0.003663$

Table 6-1 Rules of Common Logarithms (continued)

Rule	Example
3. $\log a/b = \log a - \log b$ $(a > 0, b > 0)$	$x = 478/21$ $\log x = \log 478 - \log 21$ $\log 478 = 2.6794$ $\log 21 = 1.3222$ $\log x = 1.3572$ $x = 22.76$
4. $\log a^n = n \log a$ $(a > 0, n$ is a real number$)$	$x = \sqrt[3]{374}$ $= (374)^{1/3}$ $\log x = 1/3 \log 374$ $\log 374 = 2.5729$ $\log x = 1/3(2.5729)$ $= 0.8576$ $x = 7.204$

The Characteristic

The integer or **characteristic** of the logarithm of a number is determined by the position of the decimal point in the number. The characteristic of a number can easily be found by expressing the number in scientific notation. Once in this form, the exponent is used as the characteristic.

Examples

Number	Characteristic
$3025 = 3.025 \times 10^3$	3
$302.5 = 3.025 \times 10^2$	2
$30.25 = 3.025 \times 10^1$	1
$3.025 = 3.025 \times 10^0$	0
$0.3025 = 3.025 \times 10^{-1}$	-1

Note: The characteristics of logarithms of numbers less than 1 can be written in several ways. Thus, $\log 0.0361 = \log 3.61 \times 10^{-2} = \overline{2}.5575$ (not -2.5575) or $8.5575 - 10$. Written as a negative number (as with handheld calculators) $\log 0.0361 = -1.4425$.

The Mantissa

The **mantissa** is the decimal part of the logarithm of a number. The mantissa of a series of digits is the same regardless of the position of the decimal point. Thus, the logarithms of 1.7, 17, and 170 all have the same mantissa, which is 0.230.

Antilogarithms

The number having a given logarithm is called the **antilogarithm** (antilog). The logarithm of 125 is approximately 2.0969. Therefore, the antilog of 2.0969 is $10^{2.0969}$, which is approximately 125.

Antilogs of Negative Logarithms

Using a calculator, negative logarithms can be solved simply by using the 10^x key. For example, the antilog of –2 is $10^{-2} = 0.01$. However, log and antilog tables in reference books are used with positive mantissas only. Therefore, a negative logarithm must be changed to a log with a positive mantissa to find its antilog. This change of form is accomplished by first adding and then subtracting 1, which does not alter the original value of the logarithm.

Example	
Find antilog -1.6415	
Solution	
1. Write the log as a negative characteristic minus the mantissa.	$-1.6415 = -1 - 0.6415$
2. Subtract 1 from the characteristic and add 1 to the mantissa.	$-1 - 0.6415 = -1 - 1 - 0.6415$ $+1 = -2 + 0.3585$
3. Express the result as a log having a negative characteristic and a positive mantissa.	$-2 + 0.3585 = \bar{2}.3585$
4. Use the tables to find the antilog.	antilog -1.6415 = antilog $\bar{2}.3585$ $= 0.02283$

Natural Logarithms

When a logarithmic function must be differentiated or integrated, it is convenient to rewrite the function with the number e as a base. The number e is approximately equal to 2.71828. Logarithms which have the base e are called **natural logarithms** and are denoted by ln (read: "ell-en").

$$\text{If } e^x = N, \text{ then } \log_e N = \ln N = x$$

Any number of the form a^x may be rewritten with e as the base:

$$a^x = e^{x \ln a}$$

Note: e^x is sometimes written as $\exp(x)$.

The same rules apply to natural logarithms that apply to common logarithms. See Table 6–2.

Table 6-2 Rules of Natural Logarithms

1.	$\ln ab = \ln a + \ln b$	$(a > 0, b > 0)$
2.	$\ln 1/a = -\ln a$	$(a > 0)$
3.	$\ln a/b = \ln a - \ln b$	$(a > 0, b > 0)$
4.	$\ln a^x = x \ln a$	$(a > 0, x \text{ is a real number})$
5.	$\ln e = 1$	
6.	$\ln e^x = x = e^{\ln x}$	
7.	$a^x = e^{x \ln x}$	$(a > 0)$
8.	$\ln x = (\ln 10)(\log x) = 2.3026(\log x)$	$(x > 0)$

Change of Base

Logarithms to one base can easily be changed to logarithms of another base using the following equation.

$$\log_a x = \frac{\log_b x}{\log_b a}$$

Example

$$\log_{10} x = \frac{\log_e x}{\log_e 10} = \frac{\ln x}{\ln 10}$$

$$\therefore \ \ln x = 2.302585 \log_{10} x$$

■ TRIGONOMETRY

Systems of Angular Measure

Degree

The degree is defined as 1/360 of a complete revolution.

1 revolution = 360°
1 right angle = 90°
1 degree = 60 minutes (60′)
1 minute = 60 seconds (60″)

Radian

The radian is defined as the angle subtended at the center of a circle by an arc whose length is equal to the radius of the circle. In general, an angle θ in radians is given by

$$\theta = \frac{s}{r}$$

where

s = arc length
r = radius

Relationship Between Degrees and Radians

1 revolution = 2π radians
π = 3.14159 . . .
1 degree = $2\pi/360$ radians = 0.0174.53 radian
30° = $\pi/6$ radians
45° = $\pi/4$ radians
60° = $\pi/3$ radians
90° = $\pi/2$ radians
180° = π radians

Trigonometric Functions

In trigonometry, an angle is considered positive if it is generated by a counterclockwise rotation from standard position, and negative if it is generated by a clockwise rotation (Fig. 6–2). The trigonometric functions of a positive acute angle θ can be defined as ratios of the sides of a right triangle:

$$\text{sine of } \theta = \sin \theta = y/r$$
$$\text{cosine of } \theta = \cos \theta = x/r$$
$$\text{tangent of } \theta = \tan \theta = y/x$$
$$\text{cotangent of } \theta = \cot \theta = x/y$$
$$\text{secant of } \theta = \sec \theta = r/x$$
$$\text{cosecant of } \theta = \csc \theta = r/y$$

These functions can also be expressed in terms of sine and cosine alone:

$$\tan \theta = \sin \theta/\cos \theta$$
$$\cot \theta = \cos \theta/\sin \theta$$
$$\sec \theta = 1/\cos \theta$$
$$\csc \theta = 1/\sin \theta$$

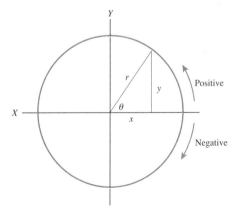

Figure 6-2 An angle is generated by rotating a ray (or half-line) about the origin of a circle. The angle is positive if it is generated by a counterclockwise rotation from the *x*-axis and negative for a clockwise rotation.

Basic Trigonometric Identities

$$\sin^2\theta + \cos^2\theta = 1$$
$$\sec^2\theta = 1 + \tan^2\theta$$

■ PROBABILITY

The **probability** of an event A is denoted $p(A)$. It is defined as follows: If an event can occur in p number of ways and can fail to occur in q number of ways, then the probability of the event occurring is $p/(p + q)$. The *odds in favor* of an event occurring are p to q.

Addition Rule

If A and B are any events, then

$$p(A \text{ or } B) = p(A) + p(B) - p(A \text{ and } B)$$

Example

The probability of drawing either a king or a black card from a deck of 52 playing cards is

$$p(\text{king or black card}) = p(\text{king}) + p(\text{black card}) - p(\text{king also black})$$
$$= 4/52 + 26/52 - 2/52$$
$$= 7/13$$

Note: If events A and B cannot occur at the same time, they are said to be mutually exclusive, and the addition rule can be simplified to

$$p(A \text{ or } B) = p(A) + p(B)$$

Multiplication Rule

If A and B are any events, then

$$p(A \text{ and } B) = p(A|B) \times p(B)$$

where

$p(A|B)$ = the probability of event A given that event B has occurred

Example

Two cards are drawn from a deck of 52 playing cards. The first card is not replaced before the second card is drawn. The probability that both cards are aces is given by

$$p(\text{both aces}) = p(\text{2nd card is ace|1st card is ace}) \times p(\text{1st card is ace})$$
$$= 3/51 \times 4/52$$
$$= 1/221$$

Notice that if the first card is an ace, $p(A|B) = 3/51$, since there are only 3 aces left of 51 remaining cards.

Note: If the occurrence of event B is in no way affected by the occurrence or nonoccurrence of event A (e.g., if the first card drawn was replaced before the second card was drawn in the preceding example), the two events are said to be independent, and the multiplication rule can be simplified to

$$p(A \text{ and } B) = p(A) \times p(B)$$

Factorial Notation(!)

A number such as $n!$ (read: n factorial) is defined by the equation

$$n! = n(n-1)(n-2) \ldots (1)$$

where

$0! = 1$ and n is a positive integer

Example

$$5! = 5 \times 4 \times 3 \times 2 \times 1 = 120$$

Permutations

Each arrangement of all or a part of a set of objects is called a **permutation**. The total number of permutations of n different objects taken r at a time is

$$_nP_r = \frac{n!}{(n-r)!}$$

Combinations

Each of the groups that can be made by taking all or a part of a set of objects, without regard to the order of arrangement of the objects in a group, is called a **combination**. The total number of combinations of n different objects taken r at a time is

$$_nC_r = \frac{n!}{r!(n - r)!}$$

■ STATISTICAL PROCEDURES

Mode

In a distribution, the numerical value that occurs most frequently is called the **mode**. While the mode is a quick and easy method of determining central tendency or "average," it is unstable (fluctuates with sample selection) and therefore has limited use.

Median

The **median** is the point on a numerical scale that has as many items above it as below it. The median is an index of "average" position in a distribution of numbers. It is insensitive to extreme values and is therefore the preferred index of central tendency when the distribution is skewed and one is interested in a "typical" value.

Mean ($\overline{X}$, μ)

The **mean** is the index of central tendency that is most often referred to as an *average*. It is more stable than the mode or median.

$$\overline{X} = \frac{\Sigma X}{n}$$

where

Σ = the sum of

X = individual raw score

n = number of scores

Note: $\overline{X}$ denotes the mean of a sample, while μ represents the mean of a population.

Standard Deviation (σ, s)

The **standard deviation** is the most widely used measure of variability (the extent to which scores deviate from each other). The equations are

$$\sigma = \sqrt{\frac{\Sigma x^2}{n}}$$ (used when finding the standard deviation of a population, with the sample taken to be population)

$$s = \sqrt{\frac{\Sigma x^2}{n-1}}$$ (used to estimate the standard deviation of a population from the sample data extracted from that population)

where

Σ = the sum of

x = deviation score (the difference between an individual score and the mean)

n = number of scores

Correlation Coefficient (Pearson r)

The **correlation coefficient** is a measure of the degree of association between two variables. The values of a correlation coefficient range from -1.0 (perfect negative or inverse relationship) through 0 (no relationship) to $+1.0$ (perfect positive or direct relationship). The higher the absolute value of the coefficient, the stronger the relationship. It should be noted that a high degree of correlation does not necessarily mean that one variable causes the other. The most commonly used correlation index, the Pearson r, can be computed as

$$r = \frac{\Sigma xy}{ns_x s_y}$$

where

r = the correlation coefficient for variables X and Y

x = deviation score for X (the difference between an individual score and the mean)

y = deviation score for Y

Σxy = sum of the products of each pair of deviation scores

n = number of X-values paired with a Y-value

s_x = standard deviation of X scores

s_y = standard deviation of Y scores

Linear Regression (Method of Least Squares)

Once a correlation has been found between two variables, it is often useful to find an equation relating them such that one variable (X) can be used to predict the second (Y). The higher the correlation between the two variables, the more accurate the prediction. The basic **linear regression equation** is a formula for making predictions about the numerical value of one variable based on the scores of another variable:

$$Y' = a + bX$$

where

Y' = a predicted value for Y

$a = \overline{Y} - b\overline{X}$

$b = \Sigma xy / \Sigma x^2$

in which

a = intercept constant

b = regression coefficient

$\overline{Y}$ = mean of variable Y

$\overline{X}$ = mean of variable X

x = deviation score for X (the difference between an individual score and the mean)

y = deviation score for Y

The graph of the linear regression equation is a straight line that "best fits" the data.

Normal Distribution Curve

The **normal distribution curve** is a symmetric, bell-shaped curve illustrating the ideal or equal distribution of continuously variable values about a population mean (see Figure 6–3). A standard normal distribution has a mean of zero and a standard deviation of one.

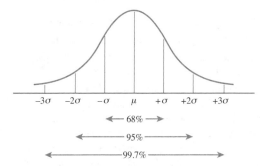

Figure 6-3 Standard deviations (σ) in a normal curve.

Percentile Rank

The **percentile rank** of a score essentially gives the percentage of the distribution that is below that score. The word *percentile* is often used to refer directly to a score in a distribution. Thus, a score with a percentile rank of 60 would be in the 60th percentile.

$$\text{percentile rank of } X = \frac{B + 1/2\,E}{n} \times 100$$

where

$B =$ the number of scores below the given score X

$E =$ the number of scores equal to the given score X

$n =$ the total number of scores

Definitions of Common Statistical Terms

Alpha (α, level of significance). The preselected level of probability that leads to rejection of the null hypothesis. It is the probability of incorrectly rejecting the null hypothesis (Type I error).

Beta (β). The probability of incorrectly accepting the null hypothesis (Type II error).

Parameter. A variable describing some characteristic of a population.

Population. An entire collection of objects as defined by a set of criteria.

Power. The power of a statistical test is the probability of correctly rejecting the null hypothesis. Numerically, power is equal to $1 - \beta$.

***P* value.** Given a test procedure and the computed value of the test statistic, the probable value or *P* value of the test is the smallest value of α that results in the rejection of the null hypothesis. Stated differently, it is the probability of an observed statistical value being equal to or greater than a given value. For example, the probability of observing a sample mean that is equal to or greater than two standard deviations away from the proposed population mean is 0.046. Thus, the smallest value of α that results in rejection of the null hypothesis (i.e., that the sample came from a population whose mean value was the proposed value) is 0.046, hence the *P* value of the observed statistic is 0.046.

Research hypothesis. A statement about the parameters of a population. A "null hypothesis" usually states that there is no difference between or among two or more populations for a given parameter. An "alternate hypothesis" usually states that there *is* a difference between or among two or more populations for a given parameter.

Sample. A subset of a population.

Statistic. A variable describing some characteristic of a sample and used to infer the same characteristic of the corresponding population.

Type I error. Rejecting the null hypothesis on the basis of a statistical test when it is actually true.

Type II error. Accepting the null hypothesis on the basis of a statistical test when it is actually false.

Universe. The group of experimental units from which a sample is selected.

Variable. A numerical quantity that can take on different values.

Reality

	Null hypothesis is true	Null hypothesis is false
Do not reject null hypothesis (non-significant result)	Correct decision probability = 1 − α	Type II error probability = β
Reject null hypothesis (significant result)	Type I error probability = α	Correct decision probability = 1 − β

Statistical Test Result

Figure 6-4 Definitions and probabilities of Type I and Type II errors.

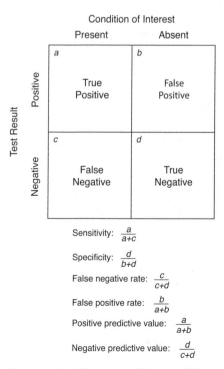

Figure 6-5 Definitions of sensitivity, specificity, and related indices.

Sensitivity. The probability that a test will be positive when the condition of interest (e.g., disease) is present.

Specificity. The probability that a test will be negative when the condition of interest (e.g., disease) is not present.

True-positive rate. Equivalent to sensitivity.

False-negative rate. The false-negatives as a percentage of all negative results.

True-negative rate. Equivalent to specificity.

False-positive rate. The false-positives as a percentage of all positive results.

Positive predictive value. The probability that the condition of interest (e.g., disease) is present when the test is positive.

Negative predictive value. The probability that the condition interest (e.g., disease) is not present when the test is negative.

■ MATHEMATICAL SIGNS AND SYMBOLS

Table 6-3

$=$	Equals
$\approx$	Equals approximately
$\neq$	Is not equal to
$\equiv$	Is identical to, is defined as
$>$	Is greater than ($\gg$ is much greater than)
$<$	Is less than ($\ll$ is much less than)
$\geq$	Is greater than or equal to (or is no less than)
$\leq$	Is less than or equal to (or is no more than)
$\pm$	Plus or minus ($\sqrt{4} = \pm 2$)
$\propto$	Is proportional to
Σ	The sum of; Σa_K means $a_1 + a_2 + \ldots + a_n$
$\bar{x}$	The average value of x
Δx	The change in x
$\dot{x}$	The derivative of x with respect to time
Π	Product of; Πa_K means $a_1 a_2 \ldots a_n$

■ THE GREEK ALPHABET

Table 6-4

Alpha	A	α	Nu	N	ν
Beta	B	β	Xi	Ξ	ξ
Gamma	Γ	γ	Omicron	O	o
Delta	Δ	δ	Pi	Π	π
Epsilon	E	ε	Rho	P	ρ
Zeta	Z	ζ	Sigma	Σ	σ
Eta	H	η	Tau	T	τ
Theta	Θ	θ	Upsilon	Υ	υ
Iota	I	ι	Phi	Φ	φ
Kappa	K	κ	Chi	X	χ
Lambda	Λ	λ	Psi	Ψ	ψ
Mu	M	μ	Omega	Ω	ω

■ RANDOM NUMBERS

A table of **random numbers** (Table 6–5) can be used to select a random sample of N items from a universe of M items using the following procedure:

Table 6-5 Random Numbers

10480	15011	01536	02011	81647	91646
22368	46573	25595	85393	30995	89189
24130	48360	22527	97265	76393	64809
42167	93093	06243	61680	07856	16376
37570	39975	81837	16656	06121	91782
77921	06907	11008	42751	27756	53498
99562	72905	56420	69994	98872	31016
96301	91977	05463	07972	18876	20922
89579	14342	63661	10281	17453	18103
85475	36857	43342	53988	53060	59533

(continued)

Table 6-5 Random Numbers (continued)

28918	69578	88231	33276	70997	79936
63553	40961	48235	03427	49626	69445
09429	93969	52636	92737	88974	33488
10365	61129	87529	85689	48237	52267
07119	97336	71048	08178	77233	13916

1. Create an arbitrary procedure for selecting entries from the table. For example, use the entries from the first line of each column.

2. Assign numbers to each of the items in the universe from 1 to M. Thus, if $M = 250$, the items would be numbered from 001 to 250 such that each item is associated with a three-digit number.

3. Decide on an arbitrary scheme for selecting digits from each entry in the table selected according to step 1. That is, each entry has five digits and for this example we need only three. Thus, we might decide to use the first, third, and fifth digits in the entry to create the required three-digit number corresponding to an item in the universe.

4. If the number formed in step 3 is $\leq M$, then the correspondingly designated item (from step 2) in the universe is selected for the random sample of N items. For example, if the first selection was the first entry in the first column of Table 6–5, 10480, the first, third, and last digits would yield the number 140. Thus, item number 140 of the universe of items would be the first picked for the sample. If a number $>M$ is formed in step 3 or is a repeated number of one already chosen, it is skipped and the next desirable number is taken. This process is continued until the random sample of N items is selected.

A widely used equation for generating random numbers is

$$x_{n+1} = \text{FRAC}\,(\pi + x_n)^5$$

The equation requires a seed number, x_n, which can be varied between 0 and 1 to give many random number sequences. The procedure for using the equation is as follows:

1. Select a number between 0 and 1 and add it to the value of π.

2. Raise the result to the fifth power.

3. Take the fraction portion (FRAC, the numbers to the right of the decimal point) as the random number.

4. Use the fraction portion of the answer as the new value of *x*.

5. Repeat the procedure until the required number of random numbers is generated.

■ SI UNITS*

"**SI units**" stands for *le Système international d'Unités,* or International System of Units. It is a system of reporting numerical values that promotes the interchangeability of information between nations and between disciplines. It consists of seven base units (Table 6–6) from which other units are derived (Table 6–7). There are two supplemental units, the *radian* for the plane angle and the *steradian* for the solid angle. The definitions of the base units are listed in the next section. Tables 6–8, 6–9, 6–10, and 6–11 contain further information on units of measurement.

Table 6-6 Base Units of SI

Physical Quantity	Base Unit	SI Symbol
Length	Meter	m
Mass	Kilogram	kg
Time	Second	s
Amount of substance	Mole	mol
Thermodynamic temperature	Kelvin	K
Electric current	Ampere	A
Luminous intensity	Candela	cd

Table 6-7 Representative Derived Units

Derived Unit	Name (Symbol)	Derivation From Base Units
Area	Square meter	m^2
Volume	Cubic meter	m^3
Force	Newton (N)	$kg \cdot m \cdot s^{-2}$
Pressure	Pascal (Pa)	$kg \cdot m^{-1} \cdot s^{-2}$ (N/m^2)
Work, energy	Joule (J)	$kg \cdot m^2 \cdot s^{-2}$ ($N \cdot m$)
Mass density	Kilogram/cubic meter	kg/m^3
Frequency	Hertz (Hz)	s^{-1}

---

*Portions of this section are reprinted with permission from *Respir Care* 33 1988:861–873.

Table 6-8 Prefixes and Symbols for Decimal Multiples and Submultiples

Factor	Prefix	Symbol
10^{18}	exa	E
10^{15}	peta	P
10^{12}	tera	T
10^9	giga	G
10^6	mega	M
10^3	kilo	k
10^2	**hecto**	**h**
10^1	**deka**	**da**
10^{-1}	**deci**	**d**
10^{-2}	**centi**	**c**
10^{-3}	milli	m
10^{-6}	micro	μ
10^{-9}	nano	n
10^{-12}	pico	p
10^{-15}	femto	f
10^{-18}	atto	a

Factors in bold do not conform to the preferred incremental changes of 10^3 and 10^{-3} but are still used outside medicine. Note that in use, they are written in plain rather than boldface type.

Table 6-9 SI Style Specifications

Specifications	Example	Incorrect Style	Correct Style
Use lowercase for symbols or abbreviations.	Kilogram	Kg	kg
Exceptions:	Kelvin	k	K
	Ampere	a	A
	Liter	l	L
Symbols are not followed by a period except at the end of a sentence.	Meter	m.	m
Do not pluralize symbols.	Kilograms	kgs	kg

(continued)

Table 6–9 SI Style Specifications (continued)

Specifications	Example	Incorrect Style	Correct Style
Names and symbols are not to be combined.	Force	kilogram · meter · s^{-2}	kg · m · s^{-2}
When numbers are printed, symbols are preferred.		100 meters 2 moles	100 m 2 mol
Use a space between the number and symbol.		50mL	50 mL
The product of units is indicated by a dot above the line.		kg × m/s^2	kg · m · s^{-2}
Use only one virgule (/) per expression.		mmol/L/s	mmol/(L · s)
Place a zero before the decimal.		.01	0.01
Decimal numbers are preferable to fractions and percents.		3/4 75%	0.75 0.75
Spaces are used to separate long numbers (optional for four-digit number).		1,500,000 1,000	1 500 000 1000 or 1 000

Table 6–10 Currently Accepted Non-SI Units

Quantity	Name	Symbol	Value in SI Units
Time	Minute	min	1 min = 60 s
	Hour	h	1 h = 60 min = 3 600 s
	Day	d	1 d = 24 h = 86 400 s
Plane angle	Degree	°	1° = (π/180) rad
	Minute	′	1′ = (1/60)° = (π/10 800) rad
	Second	″	1″ = (1/60)′ = (π/648 000) rad
Volume	Liter	L	1 L = 1 dm^3 = 10^{-3} m^3
Mass	Ton (metric)	t	1 t = 10^3 kg
Area	Hectare	ha	1 ha = 1 hm^2 = 10^4 m^2

Table 6-11 Conversion Factors for Units Commonly Used in Medicine

Physical Quantity	Conventional Unit	SI Unit	Conversion Factor*
Length	Inch (in.)	meter (m)	0.0254
	Foot (ft)	m	0.3048
Area	in.^{2}	m^2	6.452×10^{-4}
	ft^2	m^2	0.09290
Volume	dL (= 100 mL)	L	0.01
	ft^3	m^3	0.02832
	ft^3	L	28.32
	Fluid ounce → mL		29.57
Amount of substance	mg/dL	mmol/L	10/mol wt
	mEq/L	mmol/L	valence
	mL of gas at STPD	mmol	0.04462
Force	Pound (lb)	newton (N)	4.448
	Dyne	N	0.00001
	Kilogram-force	N	9.807
	Pound → kilogram-force		0.4536
	Ounce → gram-force		28.35
Pressure	cm H_2O	kilopascal (kPa)	0.09806
	mm Hg (torr)	kPa	0.1333
	Pounds/in.^{2} (psi)	kPa	6.895
	psi → cm H_2O		70.31
	cm H_2O → torr		0.736
	Standard atmosphere	kPa	101.3
	Millibar (mbar)	kPa	0.1000
Work, energy	Calorie (c)	joule (J)	4.185
	Kilocalorie (C)	J	4185
	British thermal unit (BTU)		1055
Surface tension	dyn/cm	N/m	0.001
Compliance	L/cm H_2O	L/kPa	10.20

(continued)

Table 6-11 Conversion Factors for Units Commonly Used in Medicine (continued)

Physical Quantity	Conventional Unit	SI Unit	Conversion Factor*
Resistance			
airway	cm $H_2O \cdot s \cdot L^{-1}$	kPa $\cdot s \cdot L^{-1}$	0.09806
vascular	dyn $\cdot s \cdot cm^{-5}$	kPa $\cdot s \cdot L^{-1}$	0.1000
	mm Hg $\cdot$ min $\cdot L^{-1}$	kPa $\cdot s \cdot L^{-1}$	7.998
Gas diffusion	mL $\cdot s^{-1} \cdot$ cm H_2O^{-1}	mmol $\cdot s^{-1} \cdot$ kPa^{-1}	0.4550
Gas transport	mL/min	mmol/min	0.04462
Temperature	°C	K	$K = °C + 273.15$
	°F → °C		$°C = (°F - 32)/1.8$
	°C → °F		$°F = (1.8 \cdot °C) + 32$

*To convert from conventional to SI unit, multiply conventional unit by conversion factor. To convert in the opposite direction, divide by conversion factor. Examples: 10 torr = 10 × 0.133 3 kPa = 1.333 kPa, 1 L = 1 L/0.10 = 10 dL.

■ DEFINITIONS OF BASIC UNITS

Ampere. "That constant current which, if maintained in two straight parallel conductors of infinite length, would produce between these conductors a force equal to 2×10^{-7} newton per meter of length." (CPGM, 1948)

Candela. "The luminous intensity, in the perpendicular direction, of a substance of 1/600 000 square meter of black body at the temperature of freezing platinum under a pressure of 101 325 newton per square meter." (13th CPGM, 1967)

Kelvin. "The fraction of 1/273.16 of the temperature of the triple point of water." (13th CPGM, 1967) The triple point of water is the temperature at which ice, water, and vapor coexist in equilibrium at a temperature of +0.0075°C and a pressure of 610.6 newton/m^2.

Kilogram. "Equal to the mass of the international prototype of the kilogram (held at *Sevres*)." (3rd CPGM, 1901)

Meter. "Equal to 1 650 763.73 wavelengths in vacuum of the radiation corresponding to the transition between the levels $2p_{10}$ and $5d_5$ of the krypton-86 atom." (11th CPGM*, 1960)

---

*CPGM stands for General Conference of Weights and Measures.

Mole. "The amount of substance of a system which contains as many elementary entities as there are atoms in 0.012 kilogram of carbon 12." (14th CGPM, 1971) When the mole is used, the elementary entities must be specified and may be atoms, molecules, ions, electrons, other particles, or specified groups of such particles.

Radian. The unit of measure for plane angles, defined as the angle subtended at the center of a circle by an arc whose length is equal to the radius of the circle. In general, angle (radians) = arc length/radius. Since the circumference of a circle is equal to $2 \cdot \pi$ radius of circle, a revolution of $360°$ equals $2 \cdot \pi$ radians. Radian measure is much easier to work with than degrees, minutes, and seconds, and is also more practical for use with computers.

Second. "The duration of 9 192 631 770 periods of the radiation corresponding to the transition between the two hyperfine levels of the ground state of the cesium-133 atom." (13th CPGM, 1967)

Steradian. The analogous unit of (radian) measure for solid angles. There are $4 \cdot \pi$ steradians in a sphere.

■ PHYSICAL QUANTITIES IN RESPIRATORY PHYSIOLOGY

The dimensions of the physical quantities described here are in mass/length/time units. These units provide a way of checking the validity of equations and other expressions used in the study of respiratory physiology. That is, the same mass/length/time units must be on both sides of an equation, and only identical mass/length/time units can be added or subtracted.

Volume (dimensions: length^3). Although the cubic meter (m^3) is the SI base unit for volume, the cubic decimeter (dm^3), given the name liter, has been accepted as the reference volume for stating concentrations. The cubic centimeter (cm^3) or milliliter (mL) may still be used as a volume unit other than as the denominator of a concentration unit.

According to J. F. Nunn, *Applied Respiratory Physiology*, 2nd ed. (London: Butterworths, 1978):

It is not good practice to report gas volumes under the conditions prevailing during their measurement. In the case of oxygen uptake, carbon dioxide output and the exchange of "inert" gases, we need to know the actual quantity (i.e., number of molecules) of gas exchanged and this is most conveniently expressed by stating the gas volume as it would be under standard conditions . . . (pp. 445–452)

Standard conditions are 273.15K (0°C), 101.3 kPa (760 torr) pressure, and dry (STPD). When volumes relate to anatomic measurements such as tidal volume or vital capacity, they should be expressed as they would be at body temperature and pressure, saturated (BTPS). Conversions between ambient, body, and standard conditions are made using tables or equations.

Amount of substance (dimensionless). The concentration of chemical substances is reported primarily in moles per liter (mol/L) or some multiple thereof (e.g., mmol/L). When the molecular weight of a substance is not known, the unit may be grams per liter (g/L). (Note that 1 mg/mL = 1 g/L = 1 kg/m^3.) Because water is not thought of as a chemically active substance for the purposes of humidification, it would appear that absolute humidity should still be reported in terms of weight instead of moles (i.e., mg/L). For ideal gases such as oxygen and nitrogen, 1 mole occupies 22.4 L at STPD. Therefore, the sum of the concentrations of ideal gases in a mixture would be 44.6 mmol/L.

Equivalent weights (e.g., milliequivalents) are related to molar concentrations by their ionic valence. That is, equivalent weight equals mole/valence.

Example

Thus, for example, one equivalent weight of serum calcium is 1 mole (1 gram molecular weight, 40.08 g) divided by 2 (the valence) or 20.02 equivalents. In applying this to clinical practice, we start with a normal value for calcium, which is conventionally reported as 8.8 mg/dL. First we convert to mg/L: (8.8 mg/dL) × (10 dL/L) = 88 mg/L. Next, we convert to mmol/L: (88 mg/L) × (1 mmol/40.08 mg) = 2.20 mmol/L. Serum ionized calcium (Ca^{2+}) is reported as milliequivalents per liter (mEq/L). Suppose a value for ionized calcium is reported as 2.00 mEq/L. To convert to mmol/L, (2.00 mEq/L) × (1 mmol/2 mEq) = 1.00 mmol/L. Converting the other way, (1.00 mmol/L) × (2 mEq/1 mmol) = 2.00 mEq/L. For univalent ions such as sodium, potassium, chloride, and bicarbonate, mEq/L and mmol/L are numerically equal.

Volume flow rate (dimensions: length^3 · time^{-1}). Volume flow rate is a special case of mass flow rate. We are generally interested in flow into and out of the airways and how this changes lung volume. We therefore speak of volume as if it flows—flows are expressed in liters per minute, for example. This shorthand notation overlooks an important physical fact: Gases flow; volumes do not. When we speak of a *volume flow* of so many liters per minute, what we are really saying is that the mass of gas that has exited from the lung over that time would occupy a volume of so many liters *at some specific temperature and pressure.* Thus, flow measurements require accurate temperature and pressure measurements to be accurate. Gas exchange rates should be corrected to STPD, while ventilatory gas flow rates should be corrected to BTPS. As a rule of thumb, gas volumes at STPD are about 10% less than at ATPS, while volumes at BTPS are about 10% more. Units of liters per minute (L/min), liters per second (L/s), and milliliters per minute (mL/min) are acceptable at present.

Force (dimensions: mass · length · time^{-2}). Force is defined as mass times acceleration. The SI unit of force, the newton (N), is defined as the force that will give a mass of 1 kilogram an acceleration of 1 meter per second squared (kg · m · s^{-2}).

One type of force that is in common usage is that due to gravity acting on a standard mass. This force is interpreted as *weight* (i.e., weight equals mass times acceleration due to gravity). In the British system, for example, a force of 1 pound is produced when a mass of 1 slug is accelerated at the rate of 1 foot per second per second. In the metric system, weights are often expressed in grams or kilograms. Although these units are not units of force (i.e., the weight of a 1-kg mass is 1 N), they are used as such and sometimes referred to as gram-force or kilogram-force. What is implied is that a mass of 1 gram (or kilogram) experiences a force due to standard conditions of gravity (9.8 m/s^2 or 32 ft/s^2) , or "one unit" of acceleration. Thus, 1 gram-force equals 1 gram mass times 1 unit of acceleration. This is the basis for converting pounds to kilograms and vice versa. Therefore, to say that 10 kilograms "equals" 22 pounds means that the 10-kilogram mass experiences a force of 22 pounds under standard conditions of gravity (i.e., 0.6852 slug · 32 ft · s^{-2}). At the present time, the kilogram-force is being retained as the standard unit to express weight for medical purposes.

The problem with this convention, aside from the fact that it is confusing, is that the force of gravity varies from point to point on Earth. Therefore, the weight of 1-kilogram mass, determined, for instance, with a spring scale, will vary depending on where on Earth it is measured. In space, where gravity is nil, the weight would be zero. Hence, the kilogram-force is a poor unit for standardization.

Pressure (dimensions: mass · length^{-1} · time^{-2}). In respiratory physiology, force is generally expressed as pressure, defined as force per unit area. The SI unit of force, the pascal (Pa), is defined as 1 newton per square meter (1 N/m^2). However, the pascal is inconveniently small (equivalent to about 1/10,000th of an atmosphere), so the kilopascal (kPa) has been proposed for general use in medicine. Thus, a kilopascal is about 1% of an atmosphere. A standard atmosphere is 101.3 kPa, and the partial pressure of oxygen in dry air is approximately 21 kPa. One kPa is approximately 10 centimeters of water (cm H_2O). The millimeter of mercury (mm Hg) and the centimeter of water are two gravity-based units used in medicine that will eventually be replaced for reporting gas pressures. Currently, however, medical journals are still using these units. It appears that mm Hg may be retained indefinitely for reporting blood pressure.

Work and energy (dimensions: mass · length^2 · time^{-2}). According to the work–energy theorem, the work done on a body by an applied force is equal to the change in kinetic energy of the body. Work is done when a force moves a body a given distance, or when gas is moved in response to a pressure gradient. In the SI, the unit of work is the joule (J), defined as the work done when a force of 1 newton moves a body a distance of 1 meter (i.e., 1 N · m), or when a liter of gas moves in response to a pressure gradient of 1 kilopascal (i.e., 1 L · kPa). The erg and calorie will no longer be used.

Because pressure times volume yields dimensions of energy, pressure can be interpreted as energy density (energy per unit volume). Thus, if the pressure of a system increases, it reflects a change in energy of the system, meaning that some outside agency has done work on it. When the pressure is released, useful work may be recovered. This is the principle used by air rifles and ventilators powered by compressed gas.

Power (dimensions: mass · length^2 · time^{-3}). Power is defined as the rate of change of work. The SI unit is the watt (W), defined as 1 joule per second. This unit provides a convenient link with electrical units because 1 watt equals 1 ampere times 1 volt.

Surface tension (dimensions: mass · time^{-2}). Surface tension is defined as a force per unit length existing at a liquid surface. In SI units, surface tension would be expressed as the newton per meter, which is equal to 1 Pa · m or 1 kg · s^{-2}. The unit for surface tension is likely to be called the pascal-meter. One millipascal-meter is equal to the conventional centimeter-gram-second unit (CGS) the dyne/centimeter (dyn/cm).

Compliance (dimensions: mass $\cdot$ length^{-4} $\cdot$ time^{-2}). Compliance is defined as the change in the volume of a system divided by the corresponding change in the pressure difference across the walls of the system (i.e., the slope of the pressure-volume curve). In SI units, compliance would be expressed as liter per kilopascal (L/kPa). The reciprocal, *elastance,* has units of kilopascal per liter.

Resistance (dimensions: mass $\cdot$ length^{-4} $\cdot$ time^{-1}). Resistance to laminar flow is defined as the change in the pressure difference causing flow divided by the associated change in flow rate (i.e., the slope of the flow-pressure curve). The appropriate SI units are kPa $\cdot$ L^{-1} $\cdot$ s. The reciprocal, *conductance,* has units of kPa^{-1} $\cdot$ L $\cdot$ s^{-1}.

Solubility (dimensions: time $\cdot$ length^{-1}). The solubility of a gas in liquid has been expressed in many different units. This is simplified in SI units as mmol $\cdot$ L^{1} $\cdot$ kPa^{-1}, which has been given the name *capacitance coefficient.* This coefficient varies only with temperature when a solution obeys Henry's law. For solutions with a nonlinear dissociation curve (e.g., oxygen in blood), the capacitance coefficient would be defined between two points (arterial and venous) as difference in concentration (mmol $\cdot$ L^{1}) divided by difference in partial pressure (kPa).

Temperature. Although the SI unit for temperature is the kelvin (K), some medical journals still use the Celsius scale. Temperatures expressed in degrees kelvin and Celsius both have the same-sized increments, but the kelvin scale offers the advantage of being a ratio rather than an interval scale. Thus, it has an absolute zero that makes possible statements like, "The temperature in group A was 5% higher than group B."

Reference Data

CLINICAL ABBREVIATIONS

aa	of each	nmol	nanomole
a.c.	before meals	p	after
Ad. lib.	as desired	PEEP	positive end-expiratory pressure
AG	anion gap		
Ant.	anterior	PIP	peak inspiratory pressure
ante	before	PO	by mouth
Aq.	water	PR	rectal
bid	twice daily	prn	as needed
bpm	beats per minute	pt	pint
$\bar{c}$	with	q	every
cc	cubic centimeters	qd	every day
CI	cardiac index	qh	every hour
comp	compound	q2h	every two hours
CO	cardiac output	qhs	at bedtime
DC	discontinue	qid	four times a day
dL	deciliter (= 100 mL)	qt	quart
dr	dram	$\bar{s}$	without
g	gram	SI	stroke index
gtt	drop	sol	solution
kg	kilogram	stat	immediately
μg	microgram	STP	standard temperature and pressure
mEq	milliequivalent		
mg	milligram	tid	three times daily
mL	milliliter	vol%	volume percent

■ PHYSIOLOGICAL ABBREVIATIONS

The terminology and abbreviations listed here are those suggested by the American College of Chest Physicians and the American Thoracic Society Joint Committee.

X_A or Xa	A small capital letter or lowercase letter on the same line following a primary symbol is a qualifier to further define the primary symbol. When small capital letters are not available, large capital letters may be used as subscripts, e.g., $X_A = X_A$.
ATPD	Ambient temperature and pressure, dry
ATPS	Ambient temperature and pressure, saturated with water vapor at these conditions
B	Barometric (qualifying symbol)
BTPS	Body conditions: body temperature, ambient pressure, and saturated with water vapor at these conditions
C	A general symbol for compliance; volume change per unit of applied pressure; concentration
c	Capillary
c'	Pulmonary end capillary
C/V_L	Specific compliance
CD	Cumulative inhalation dose. The total dose of an agent inhaled during bronchial challenge testing; it is the sum of the products of concentration multiplied by the number of breaths at that concentration.
Cdyn	Dynamic compliance: compliance measured at point of zero gas flow at the mouth during active breathing. The respiratory frequency should be designated; e.g., Cdyn 40.
C_{st}	Static compliance; compliance determined from measurements made during conditions of prolonged interruption of airflow
D/V_A	Diffusion per unit of alveolar volume
Dk	Diffusion coefficient or permeability constant as described by Krogh; it equals $D \cdot (P_B - P_{H_2O})/V_A$
Dm	Diffusing capacity of the alveolar capillary membrane (STPD)

Dx (e.g., DLco)   Diffusing capacity of the lung expressed as volume (STPD) of gas (x) uptake per unit alveolar capillary pressure difference for the gas used. Unless otherwise stated, carbon monoxide is assumed to be the test gas, i.e., D is Dco. A modifier can be used to designate the technique, e.g., Dsb is single-breath carbon monoxide diffusing capacity and Dss is steady-state carbon monoxide diffusing capacity. (*Author's note:* This recommendation has not been widely accepted. DL_{co}, $DL_{co}SB$, and $DL_{co}SS$ are still the most commonly used abbreviations.)

E   Expired (qualifying symbol)

ERV   Expiratory reserve volume; the maximum volume of air exhaled from the end-expiratory level

est   Estimated

f   Ventilator frequency

f_b Breathing frequency

F   Fractional concentration of a gas

FEFmax   The maximum forced expiratory flow achieved during the FVC

$FEF_{25\%-75\%}$ Mean forced expiratory flow during the middle half of the FVC (formerly called the maximum mid-expiratory flow rate)

$FEF_{75\%}$ Instantaneous forced expiratory flow after 75% of the FVC has been exhaled

$FEF_{200-1200}$ Mean forced expiratory flow between 200 mL and 1200 mL of the FVC (formerly called the maximum expiratory flow rate)

FEF_x Forced expiratory flow, related to some portion of the FVC curve. Modifiers refer to the amount of the FVC already *exhaled* when the measurement is made.

FET_x The forced expiratory time for a specified portion of the FVC; e.g., $FET_{95\%}$ is the time required to deliver the first 95% of the FVC and $FET_{25\%-75\%}$ is the time required to deliver the $FEF_{25\%-75\%}$

FEV   Forced expiratory volume

FEV/FVC%   Forced expiratory volume (timed) to forced vital capacity ratio, expressed as a percentage

FIF_x	Forced inspiratory flow. As in the case of the FEF, the appropriate modifiers must be used to designate the volume at which flow is being measured. Unless otherwise specified, the volume qualifiers indicate the volume inspired from RV at the point of the measurement.
FRC	Functional residual capacity; the sum of RV and ERV (the volume of air remaining in the lungs at the end-expiratory position). The method of measurement should be indicated, as with RV.
FVC	Forced vital capacity
Gaw	Airway conductance, the reciprocal of Raw
Gaw/V_L	Specific conductance, expressed per liter of lung volume at which G is measured (also referred to as sGaw)
I	Inspired (qualifying symbol)
IRV	Inspiratory reserve volume; the maximum volume of air inhaled from the end-inspiratory level
IC	Inspiratory capacity; the sum of IRV and V_T
L	Lung (qualifying symbol)
max	Maximum
MIP	Maximum inspiratory pressure
MEP	Maximum expiratory pressure
MVV_x	Maximum voluntary ventilation. The volume of air expired in a specified period during repetitive maximum respiratory effort. The respiratory frequency is indicated by a numerical qualifier; e.g., MVV_{60} is MW performed at 60 breaths per minute. If no qualifier is given, an unrestricted frequency is assumed.
OI	Oxygenation index
p	Physiologic
P	Pressure, blood or gas
PA	Pulmonary artery
Paw	Airway pressure
PD	Provocative dose; the dose of an agent used in bronchial challenge testing that results in a defined change in a specific physiologic parameter. The parameter tested and the percent change in this parameter is expressed in cumulative

	dose units over the time following exposure that the positive response occurred. For example, $PD_{35}sGaw = x$ units/y minutes, where x is the cumulative inhalation dose and y the time at which a 35% fall in sGaw was noted.
PEF	Peak expiratory flow: the highest forced expiratory flow measured with a peak flowmeter
pred	Predicted
P_{st}	Static transpulmonary pressure at a specified lung volume; e.g., $P_{st}TLC$ is static recoil pressure measured at TLC (maximal recoil pressure)
Q	Volume of blood
Q_c	Capillary blood volume (usually expressed as V_c in the literature, a symbol inconsistent with those recommended for blood volumes). When determined from the following equation, Q_c represents the effective pulmonary capillary blood volume, that is, capillary blood volume in intimate association with alveolar gas: $1/D = 1/D_m + 1/(\Theta \cdot Q_c)$.
Raw	Airway resistance
rb	Rebreathing
RQ	Respiratory quotient
R_{us}	Resistance of the airways on the alveolar side (upstream) of the point in the airways where intraluminal pressure equals intrapleural pressure, measured under conditions of maximum expiratory flow
RV	Residual volume; that volume of air remaining in the lungs after maximum exhalation. The method of measurement should be indicated in the test or, when necessary, by appropriate qualifying symbols.
SBN	Single-breath nitrogen test; a test in which plots of expired nitrogen concentration versus expired volume after inspiration of 100% oxygen are recorded. The closing volume and slope of phase III are two parameters measured by this test.
STPD	Standard conditions: temperature 0°C, pressure 760 mm Hg, and dry (0 water vapor)
t	Time (qualifying symbol)
T	Tidal
TGV	Thoracic gas volume; the volume of gas within the thoracic cage as measured by body plethysmography

TLC	Total lung capacity; the sum of all volume compartments or the volume of air in the lungs after maximal inspiration. The method of measurement should be indicated, as with RV.
V	Gas volume. The particular gas as well as its pressure, water vapor conditions, and other special conditions must be specified in text or indicated by appropriate qualifying symbols.
v	Venous
$\bar{v}$	Mixed venous
$\dot{V}A$	Alveolar ventilation per minute (BTPS)
$\dot{V}CO_2$	Carbon dioxide production per minute (STPD)
$\dot{V}D$	Ventilation per minute of the physiologic dead space (wasted ventilation), BTPS, defined by the following equation: $$\dot{V}D = \dot{V}E(PaCO_2 - PECO_2/(PaCO_2 - PICO_2)$$
VD	The physiologic dead-space volume defined as $\dot{V}D/f$
VDan	Volume of the anatomic dead space (BTPS)
$\dot{V}E$	Expired volume per minute (BTPS)
$\dot{V}I$	Inspired volume per minute (BTPS)
Viso$\dot{V}$	Volume of isoflow; the volume when the expiratory flow rates become identical when flow-volume loops performed after breathing room air and helium–oxygen mixtures are compared
$\dot{V}O_2$	Oxygen consumption per minute (STPD)
$\dot{V}$max X	Forced expiratory flow, related to the total lung capacity or the actual volume of the lung at which the measurement is made. *Modifiers (X) refer to the amount of the lung volume remaining when the measurement is made.* For example, $\dot{V}$max 75% is instantaneous forced expiratory flow when the lung is at 75% of its TLC. $\dot{V}$max 3.0 is instantaneous forced expiratory flow when the lung volume is 3.0 L. [*Author's note:* It is still common to find reports in which modifiers refer to the amount of VC remaining.]
V_T	Tidal volume; TV is also commonly used

■ BLOOD-GAS MEASUREMENTS

Abbreviations for these values are readily composed by combining the general symbols recommended earlier. The following are examples:

Pa_{CO_2}	Arterial carbon dioxide tension
P_{O_2}	Partial pressure of oxygen
F_{IO_2}	Fraction of inspired air
P_A	Alveolar pressure
V_A	Alveolar volume
$C(a-v)_{O_2}$	Arteriovenous oxygen content difference
Cc'_{O_2}	Oxygen content of pulmonary end capillary blood
F_{ECO}	Fractional concentration of carbon dioxide in expired gas
$P(A-a)_{O_2}$	Alveolar–arterial oxygen pressure difference; the previously used symbol, $A-aD_{O_2}$, is not recommended.
Sa_{O_2}	Arterial oxygen saturation of hemoglobin
$\dot{Q}_S$	Physiologic shunt flow (total venous admixture) as a fraction of total blood flow ($\dot{Q}_T$) defined by the following equation when gas and blood data are collected during ambient air breathing:

$$\dot{Q}_S = \frac{Cc'_{O_2} - Ca_{O_2}}{Cc'_{O_2} - C\bar{v}_{O_2}} \cdot Q_T$$

P_{ETO_2}	P_{O_2} of end-tidal expired gas
F_{CO_2}	Fractional concentration of oxygen
R	A general symbol for resistance, pressure per unit flow
R_E	Respiratory exchange ratio
REE	Resting energy expenditure
S	Saturation in the blood phase
sat	Saturated
sGaw	Specific airway conductance
S_{O_2}	Oxygen saturation
T	Temperature
TCT	Total cycle time
T_E	Expiratory time
T_I	Inspiratory time
VC	Vital capacity

■ BASIC PHARMACOLOGICAL FORMULAS AND DEFINITIONS

Solutions: Definitions and Terms

Solution: a homogeneous mixture (usually liquid) of the molecules, atoms, or ions of two or more different substances.

Solute: the dissolved substance (which may be a gas, liquid, or solid) in a solution.

Solvent: the dissolving medium in a solution.

Isotonic solutions: solutions having equal osmotic pressure.

Buffer solutions: aqueous solution able to resist changes of pH with addition of acid or base.

Gram molecular weight: the *atomic weight* of a compound expressed in grams. The gram molecular weight (formula weight) is the weight of a mole of the substance.

Equivalent weight: the weight of a substance that either receives or donates 1 mole of electrons. One gram equivalent weight of any electrolyte has the same chemical combining power as 1 gram of hydrogen. The equivalent weight of a substance is calculated by the equation:

$$\text{Equivalent weight} = \frac{\text{gram molecular weight}}{\text{valence}}$$

Milliequivalent (mEq): one-thousandth of an equivalent weight.

Normal solution: 1 gram equivalent weight of solute per liter of solution. This should not be confused with the term "normal saline," which is used to designate a solution that is isotonic with human body fluid. Normal saline is a 0.9% solution of sodium chloride or 9 g per 1,000 mL.

Molar solution: 1 mole of solute per liter of solution.

Molal solution: 1 mole of solute per 1,000 grams of solvent.

Osmole solution: molarity × number of particles per molecule.

Osmolar solution: 1 osmole per liter of solution. The osmolality of extracellular fluid can be calculated according to the formula

$$\text{serum osmolality (mOsm/kg)} = 2 \times \text{Na (mEq/L)} + \frac{\text{glucose (mg/dL)}}{18}$$

$$+ \frac{\text{BUN (mg/dL)}}{2.8} + \frac{\text{ETOH (mg/dL)}}{4.6} + \frac{\text{isopropanolol (mg/dL)}}{6}$$

$$+ \frac{\text{methanol (mg/dL)}}{3.2} + \frac{\text{ethylene glycol (mg/dL)}}{6.2}$$

Drug Dosage Calculation

Calculating Dosages from Stock Solutions, Tablets, or Capsules

1. Convert all measurements to the same unit.
2. Set up the following proportion:

$$\frac{\text{Original drug strength}}{\text{Amount supplied}} = \frac{\text{Prescribed dosage}}{\text{Unknown amount to be supplied}}.$$

3. Calculate the dosage.

Example

Your patient is going to surgery. She weighs 60 kg, and the physician ordered 0.02 mg/kg of atropine preoperatively. You only have tablets of 0.4 mg/tablet strength. How many tablets do you give the patient?

Original drug strength = 0.4 mg
Amount supplied = 1 tablet
Prescribed dosage = 0.02 mg/kg $\times$ 60 kg = 1.2 mg
Amount to be given = x

Using the above formula, we get

$$\frac{0.4 \text{ mg}}{1 \text{ tablet}} = \frac{1.2 \text{ mg}}{x \text{ tablets}}$$

$$0.4x = 1.2$$

$$x = 1.2/0.4 = 3 \text{ tablets}.$$

Calculating Dosages from Percent-Strength Solutions

Types of Percentage Preparations

Weight to weight: the number of grams of active ingredient in 100 g of a mixture.

Weight to volume: the number of grams of active ingredient in 100 mL of a mixture.

Volume to volume: the number of milliliters of active ingredient in 100 mL of a mixture.

1. When preparing percentage solutions, the following rule applies:

     A 1.0% solution contains 1.0 g in 100 mL.

     A 0.1% solution contains 0.1 g in 100 mL. This is based on the fact that 1.0 mL of H_2O at STP has a mass of 1.0 g (Table A-1).

2. Calculate the weight strength.

Table A-1 Percentage Concentrations of Solutions[*]

Percentages	Ratio	g/mL	mg/mL
100	1:1	1	1000
10	1:10	0.1	100
5	1:20	0.05	50
1	1:100	0.01	10
0.5	1:200	0.005	5
0.1	1:1,000	0.001	1

[*]Weight to volume.

Example

How much isuprel is delivered in an aerosol composed of 0.5 mL 1:200 isoproterenol (Isuprel) in 3.0 mL of saline?

Answer

A 1:200 solution contains 5 mg of drug per mL. Thus, 0.5 ml of a 1:200 (weight to volume) solution contains 0.5 mL × 5 mg/mL = 2.5 mg of drug. Therefore, the aerosol contains 2.5 mg of isoproterenol in a total of 3.5 mL of solution (0.5 mL isoproterenol + 3.0 mL saline, which is a 1:6 volume to volume ratio).

Unfortunately, the "ratio by simple parts" prescription still persists. For instance, a physician may order aerosol therapy with a 1:8 solution of isoetharine. This indicates one part medication to eight parts diluent. However, this type of prescription does not specify the actual dosage of isoetharine (either volume or weight) or the units, although usually milliliters is assumed.

■ MISCELLANEOUS REFERENCE DATA

Table A-2 Measurement Units

The Apothecary System	The Avoirdupois System
Weight	*Weight*
20 grains = 1 scruple	437.5 grains = 1 ounce
3 scruples = 1 dram	16 ounces = 1 pound
8 drams = 1 ounce	7,000 grains = 1 pound
12 ounces = 1 pound	
Volume	
60 minims = 1 fluid dram	
8 fluid drams = 1 fluid ounce	
16 fluid ounces = 1 pint	
2 pints = 1 quart	
4 quarts = 1 gallon	

Table A-3 Approximate Conversion Equivalents

Liquid		
Metric	Apothecary	Household
1 liter (1000 mL)	1 quart (2 pints)	2 tumblerfuls
500 milliliters (mL)	1 pint (16 fluid ounces)	3 teacupfuls
360 mL	12 fluid ounces (1 pound)	2 teacupfuls
30 mL	1 ounce (8 drams)	2 tablespoonfuls
4 mL	1 dram (60 minims)	1 small teaspoonful
1 mL	16 minims	1/4 teaspoonful
0.06 mL	1 minim	1 drop
Weight		
Metric	Apothecary	Avoirdupois
1 kilogram (1000 grams)	–	2.2 pounds
500 grams	7680 grains	–
454 grams	5760 grains	1 pound (16 ounces)
29 grams	480 grains	1 ounce (437 grains)
4 grams	60 grains	–

Table A-3 Approximate Conversion Equivalents (continued)

Weight		
Metric	Apothecary	Avoirdupois
1 gram (1000 mg)	15 grains	–
60 milligrams (mg)	1 grain	1 grain
1 mg (1000 micrograms)	1/60 grains	–

Table A-4 Deposition of Aerosol Particles (Mouth Breathing)

Particle Size (μm)	Maximum Retention (%)	Site of Retention
>10	100	Pharynx, larynx, trachea
5	90-95	Larynx, bronchi, bronchioles
3	8.5	Bronchioles, acini
1	60	Acini
0.6	35	Alveoli (>60% may be exhaled)
<0.1	(0)	Evaporate or coalesce

Table A-5 Physical Factors in Aerosol Deposition

Factor	Size/Type Particle	Site of Deposition	Remarks
Inertial impaction	High density > 10 μm	Nose, mouth, pharynx, larynx, airway bifurcations	Increased with high flow rate
Sedimentation (gravity)	High density 1-6 μm	Bronchioles, acini	Increased with deep, slow breathing
Diffusion	<1 μm	Entire pulmonary tree, acini, alveoli	Increased with breath-holding

Table A-6 Conversion Table for Temperature[*]

°C	°F	°C	°F	°C	°F	°C	°F
15	59.0	26	78.8	37	98.6	48	118.4
16	60.8	27	80.6	38	100.4	49	120.2
17	62.6	28	82.4	39	102.2	50	122.0
18	64.4	29	84.2	40	104.0	51	123.8
19	66.2	30	86.0	41	105.8	52	125.6
20	68.0	31	87.8	42	107.6	53	127.4
21	69.8	32	89.6	43	109.4	54	129.2
22	71.6	33	91.4	44	111.2	55	131.0
23	73.4	34	93.2	45	113.0	56	132.8
24	75.2	35	95.0	46	114.8	57	134.6
25	77.0	36	96.8	47	116.6	58	136.4

[*]To convert Celsius to Fahrenheit:	To convert Fahrenheit to Celsius:
1. Multiply by 1.8	1. Subtract 32.
2. Add 32.	2. Divide by 1.8

Celsius		*Fahrenheit*
0	Water freezes	32
22	Room temp.	72
37	Body temp.	98.6
100	Water boils	212
121	Autoclave temp.	250

Table A-7 Conversion Table for Volume

Volume	cc	In.^{3}	fl oz	Quarts	Liters
1 cc	1.00	0.061	0.0338	0.001057	0.00100
1 in.^{3}	16.39	1.00	0.554	0.0173	0.01639
1 fl oz	29.6	1.804	1.00	0.03125	0.0296
1 quart	946	57.75	32.0	1.00	0.946
1 liter	1000	61.0	33.8	1.056	1.00

Table A-8 Conversion Table for Weight

Weight	gr	g	lb	kg
1 grain (gr)	1.00	0.0648	0.0001429	0.0000648
1 gram (g)	15.43	1.00	0.002205	0.001000
1 pound (lb)	7000	454	1.00	0.454
1 kilogram (kg)	15432	1000	2.205	1.00

Table A-9 Conversion Table for Length

Length	cm	in.	ft	yd	m
1 centimeter	1.00	0.394	00328	0.01094	0.0100
1 inch	2.54	1.00	0.0833	0.0278	0.0254
1 foot	30.48	12.0	1.00	0.333	0.305
1 yard	91.4	36.0	3.00	1.00	0.914
1 meter	100.0	39.4	3.28	1.094	1.00
1 kilometer	100,000	39,400	3280	1094	1000
1 mile	160,903	63,360	5280	1760	1609

Table A-10 Conversion Table for Pressure

Known Value	in. H_2O	in. Hg	psi	cm H_2O	mm Hg	atm	mbar	Pa	kPa
Inch of water* (H_2O)	1.000	0.074	0036	2.540	1.868	0.002	2.491	249.1	0.249
Inch of mercury (Hg)**	13.59	1.000	0.491	34.53	25.40	0.033	33.86	3386	3.386
Pound/inch² (psi)	27.68	2.036	1.000	70.31	51.72	0.068	68.95	6895	6.895
Centimeter of water (cm H_2O)	0.394	0.029	0.014	1.000	0.736	0.001	0.981	98.06	0.098
Millimeter of mercury (mm Hg)	0.535	0.039	0.019	1.360	1.000	0.001	1.333	133.3	0.133
Atmosphere, standard (atm)	406.8	29.92	14.70	1033	760.0	1.000	1013	101325	101.3
Millibar (mbar)	0.401	0.030	0.014	1.020	0.750	0.001	1.000	100.0	0.100
Pascal, newton/m² (Pa)	0.004	0.0003	0.0001	0.010	0.008	10^{-5}	0.010	1.000	0.001
Kilopascal (kPa)	4.015	0.295	0.145	10.20	7.501	0.010	10.00	1000	1.000

*Water at 39.2°F (4°C).
**Mercury at 32°F (0°C).
To convert: Multiply *known value* by appropriate *conversion factor*. Example: To convert 100 in. of water to cm H_2O, multiply 100 by 2.540 = 254 cm H_2O.

Table A-11 Conversion Table for Tubes/Catheters

French	Approximate Millimeters (ID)*	Outside Diameter (OD)*	
		Inches	Millimeters
6	1.0	0.079	2
8	1.5	0.105	2.7
10	2.0	0.131	3.3
12	2.5	0.158	4
14	3.0	0.184	4.7
16	3.5	0.210	5.3
18	4.0	0.236	6
20	4.5	0.263	6.7
22	5.0	0.288	7.3
24	5.5	0.315	8
26	6.0	0.341	8.7
28	6.5	0.367	9.3
30	7.0	0.398	10
32	7.5	0.420	10.7
34	8.0	0.446	11.3

*ID = inside diameter; OD = outside diameter.

Table A-12 Conversion Table for Hypodermic Needle Tubing

Gauge	Inches (OD)	Inches (ID)
12	0.109	0.085
14	0.083	0.063
16	0.065	0.047
18	0.050	0.033
19	0.042	0.027
20	0.035	0.023
21	0.032	0.020
22	0.028	0.016
23	0.025	0.013
24	0.022	0.012
25	0.020	0.010
26	0.018	0.010
28	0.014	0.007
30	0.012	0.006
32	0.009	0.004

Table A-13 Average Body Surface Area (BSA) to Age, Weight, and Height

Age	Height (in.)	Weight (lb)	BSA (m^2)
Newborn	20	6.6	0.20
3 mo	21	11.0	0.25
1 yr	31	22.0	0.45
3 yr	38	32.0	0.62
6 yr	48	46.0	0.80
9 yr	53	66.0	1.05
15 yr	63	110.0	1.50
Adult	68	154.0	1.75

Table A-14 Body Surface Area (BSA) Prediction Equations[*]

Infant (2.5-20 kg)

$BSA (m^2) = (3.6 wt + 9)/100$

Child (20-40 kg)

$BSA (m^2) = (2.5 wt + 33)/100$

General (Dubois)

$BSA (m^2) = wt^{0.425} \times ht^{0.725} \times 0.00781$

[*]Weight in kg, height in cm.

Table A-15 Pediatric Body Surface Area (BSA) Chart

Infant		Child	
Weight (kg)	BSA (m^2)	Weight (kg)	BSA (m^2)
3	0.20	20	0.83
4	0.23	22	0.88
5	0.27	24	0.93
6	0.31	26	0.98
7	0.34	28	1.03
6	0.31	30	1.08
9	0.41	32	1.13
10	0.45	34	1.18
11	0.49	36	1.23
12	0.52	38	1.28
13	0.56	40	1.33
14	0.59		
15	0.63		
16	0.67		
17	0.70		
18	0.74		
19	0.77		
20	0.81		

Table A-16 1983 Metropolitan Life Insurance Height and Weight Tables*

Men			
Height ft in. (cm)	Small Frame lb (kg)	Medium Frame lb (kg)	Large Frame lb (kg)
5′ 2″	128-134	131-141	138-150
(157)	(58-61)	(60-64)	(63-68)
5′ 4″	132-138	135-145	142-156
(163)	(60-63)	(61-66)	(65-71)
5′ 6″	136-142	139-151	146-164
(168)	(62-65)	(63-69)	(66-75)
5′ 8″	140-148	145-157	152-172
(173)	(64-67)	(66-71)	(69-78)
5′ 10″	144-154	151-163	158-180
(178)	(65-70)	(69-74)	(72-82)
6′ 0″	149-160	157-170	164-188
(183)	(68-73)	(71-77)	(75-85)
6′ 2″	155-168	164-178	172-197
(188)	(70-76)	(75-81)	(78-90)
6′ 4″	162-172	171-187	181-207
(193)	(74-78)	(78-85)	(82-94)

Women			
Height ft in. (cm)	Small Frame lb (kg)	Medium Frame lb (kg)	Large Frame lb (kg)
4′ 10″	102-111	109-121	118-131
(147)	(46-50)	(50-55)	(54-60)
5′ 0″	104-115	113-126	122-137
(152)	(47-52)	(51-57)	(55-62)
5′ 2″	108-121	118-132	128-143
(157)	(49-055)	(54-60)	(58-65)
5′ 4″	114-127	124-138	134-151
(163)	(52-058)	(056-63)	(61-69)

Table A-16 1983 Metropolitan Life Insurance Height and Weight Tables* (continued)

Women			
Height ft in. (cm)	Small Frame lb (kg)	Medium Frame lb (kg)	Large Frame lb (kg)
5' 6"	120-133	130-144	140-159
(168)	(55-60)	(59-65)	(64-72)
5' 8"	126-139	136-150	146-167
(173)	(57-63)	(62-68)	(66-76)
5' 10"	132-145	142-156	152-173
(178)	(60-66)	(65-71)	(69-79)
6' 0"	138-151	148-162	158-179
(183)	(63-69)	(67-74)	(72-81)

*In shoes with 1-in. heels and clothes weighing approximately 5 lb.

Table A-17 Comparative Nomenclature of Bronchopulmonary Anatomy

Jackson-Huber	Number (Color) Key to Petit Reviews		Boyden	Brock	Thoracic Society of Great Britain
Right Upper lobe					
Apical	1	(Red)	B^1	Apical	Apical
Anterior	2	(Light blue)	B^2	Pectoral	Anterior
Posterior	3	(Green)	B^3	Subapical	Posterior
Right middle lobe					
Lateral	4^R	(Purple)	B^4	Lateral	Lateral
Medial	5^R	(Orange)	B^5	Medial	Medial
Right lower lobe					
Superior	6	(Lavender)	B^6	Apical	Apical
Medial basal	7	(Olive)	B^7	Cardiac	Medial basal
Anterior basal	8	(Yellow)	B^8	Anterior basal	Anterior basal
Lateral basal	9	(Red)	B^9	Middle basal	Lateral basal

(continued)

Table A-17 Comparative Nomenclature of Bronchopulmonary Anatomy (continued)

Jackson–Huber	Number (Color) Key to Petit Reviews		Boyden	Brock	Thoracic Society of Great Britain
Posterior basal	10	(Turquoise)	B^{10}	Posterior basal	Posterior basal
Left upper lobe					
Upper division	1-3	(Red)			Upper division
Apical-posterior			$B^{1\&3}$	Apical and subapical	Apicoposterior or apical and posterior
Anterior	2	(Light blue)	B^2	Pectoral	Anterior
Lower (lingular division)					
Superior lingular	4^L	(Purple)	B^4	Superior lingular	Superior lingular
Inferior lingular	5^L	(Orange)	B^5	Inferior lingular	Inferior lingular
Left lower lobe					
Superior	6	(Lavender)	B^6	Apical	Apical
Anteromedial	8	(Yellow)	$B^{7\&8}$	Anterior	Anterior basal
Lateral basal	9	(Red)	B^9	Middle basal	Lateral basal
Posterior basal	10	(Turquoise)	B^{10}	Posterior basal	Posterior basal

Table A-18 Incubator Temperatures According to Age

Age (day)	Birth Weight <1500 g		Birth Weight >1500 g		Birth Weight >2500 g and Gestation >36 wk	
	°C	°F	°C	°F	°C	°F
1st	34.3	93.8	33.4	92.1	33.0	91.4
2nd	33.7	92.7	32.7	90.9	32.4	90.4
3rd	33.5	92.3	32.4	90.4	31.9	89.4
4th	33.5	92.3	32.3	90.2	31.5	88.6
6th	33.5	92.3	32.1	89.8	30.9	87.6
8th	33.5	92.3	32.1	89.8	30.6	87.0
10th	33.5	92.3	32.1	89.8	30.2	86.4
12th	33.5	92.3	32.1	89.8	29.5	85.1
14th	33.4	92.1	32.1	89.8	–	–

Table A-19 Airway and Alveolar Dimensions from Birth to Adult

Age	Trachea		Bronchus		
	Length (mm)	Diameter (mm)	Length (mm)	Diameter (mm)	Number of Alveoli
Birth	40	6	9	5.0	24×10^6
1 yr	43	7.8	11	6.3	129×10^6
5 yr	56	10	13.5	7.5	250×10^6
10 yr	63	11	14.7	8.6	280×10^6
16 yr	74	14	20	10.0	290×10^6
Adult	90-150	14-18	22	12.7	296×10^6

Table A-20 Approximate Daily Requirements of Calories and Water

Age (yr)	Calories (kg)	Water (mL/kg)
Infancy	110	150
1-3	100	125
4-6	90	100
7-9	80	75
10-12	70	75
13-15	60	50
16-19	50	50
Adult	40	50

Table A-21 Capabilities of Disinfecting Agents Commonly Used in Respiratory Care[*]

Disinfectant	Gram-Positive Bacteria	Gram-Negative Bacteria	Tubercle Bacillus	Spores	Viruses	Fungi
Soaps	0	0	0	0	0	0
Detergents	±	≠	0	0	0	0
Quaternary ammonium compounds	+	±	0	0	±	±
Acetic acid	?	+	?	?	?	±
Alcohols	+	+	+	0	±	±
Hot water (<100°C)	+	+	+	±	±	?
Glutaraldehydes	+	+	+	±	+	+
Hydrogen peroxide-based compounds	+	+	+	±	+	+
Steam (>100°C)	+	+	+	+	+	+
Ethylene oxide	+	+	+	+	+	+

[*] + = good; ± = fair; ≠ = poor; ? = unknown; 0 = little or none.

Table A-22 Variables and Calculated Parameters for Characterizing Nebulizer Performance

Variable	Symbol	Primary Measured Variable or Equation
Output Flow	OF	Primary measured variable
Initial Charge	IC	Primary measured variable
Retained Charge	RC	Primary measured variable
Inhaled Aerosol	IA	Primary measured variable
Lung Deposition	LD	Primary measured variable
Output Aerosol	OA	$OA = IC - RC$
Output Rate	OR	$OR = \dfrac{OA}{NT}$
Inhaled Aerosol Rate	IAR	$IAR = \dfrac{IA}{NT}$
Wasted Aerosol	WA	$WA = OA - IA = IC - RC - IA$
Exhaled Aerosol	EA	$EA = IA - LD$
Nebulizer Efficiency	NE	$NE = \dfrac{OA}{IC}$
Conserver Efficiency	CE	$CE = \dfrac{SE}{NE} - BE = \dfrac{IA}{OA} - BE = DE - BE$

(continued)

Table A-22 Variables and Calculated Parameters for Characterizing Nebulizer Performance (continued)

Variable	Symbol	Primary Measured Variable or Equation
Breathing Efficiency (assuming sinusoidal flow and CE = 0, see Appendix)	BE	$BE = \dfrac{IA}{OA} = \dfrac{f \times \left(\left(\left(-V_T \cos\left(\sin^{-1}\left(\dfrac{OF}{\pi f V_T} \right) \right) \right) + V_T + OF \times \left(\dfrac{1}{2f} - \left(\dfrac{\sin^{-1}\left(\dfrac{OF}{\pi f V_T} \right)}{\pi f} \right) \right) \right)}{OF}$
Retention Efficiency	RE	$RE = \dfrac{LD}{IA}$
System Efficiency	SE	$SE = (CE + BE) \times NE = DE \times NE = \dfrac{IA}{IC}$
Delivery Efficiency	DE	$DE = \dfrac{SE}{NE} = \dfrac{IA}{IC} \times \dfrac{IC}{OA} = \dfrac{IA}{OA} = CE + BE$
Treatment Efficiency	TE	$TE = \dfrac{LD}{IC} = \dfrac{LD}{IA} \times \dfrac{IA}{IC} = RE \times SE$

TRANSLATION OF COMMONLY USED WORDS

Table A-23 French Words

English	French	Approximate Phonetic Pronunciation
Baby	Bébé	Bay-Bay
Bed	Lit	Lee
Blood	Sang	Sahng
Breath	Souffle	Sufl
Breathe	Respirer	Res-peer'-ay
Cannula	Canule	Ka'-nuel
Chest	Thoracique	Thor-a-'seek
Cough (n)	Toux	Too
Deep	Profond	Pro-fond'
Disease	Maladie	Mal-a-dee
Doctor	Docteur	Dock-'tœr
Down	En bas	Abn-'bah
Family	Famille	Fahm-'eey-uh
Fast	Rapide	Rah-'peed
Head	Tête	Teht
Heart	Coeur	Ker
Hood	Coiffe	Kwaff
In	En	Ahn
Intensive Care Unit	Unite de Soins Intensifs	Uni-'tay duh Swähnzan-tawn-zeef
Lay	Poser	Poz-ay
Left	Gauche	Gōsh
Listen to	Écouter	Ay-coo'-tay
Lungs	Poumon	Poo-'mahn
Mask	Masque	Mahsk
Mechanical ventilation	Respiration assistee	Reh-spee-rah-see-awn ah see'-stay
Medication	Médication	May-dee-'cah-see-awn

(continued)

Table A-23 French Words (continued)

English	French	Approximate Phonetic Pronunciation
Mist	Brume	Bruem
Mouth	Bouche	Boosh
Mucous	Mucus	Mew-'kus
Name	Nom	Noh
Needle	Aiguille	Ay-'gee-yah
No	Non	Noh
No smoking	Défense de fumer	Duh-'fonce duh foo-'may
Normal	Normal	Normal
Nose	Nez	Nay
Nurse (female)	Infirmière	An-'firm-ee-'air
Out	Hors	Or
Oxygen	Oxygène	Oxy-'jehn
Oxygen tent	Tente à oxygene	Tahnt-'à oxy-'jehn
Pain	Douleur	Doo-'lure
Patient	Patient	Pa-'see-ahn
Position	Position	Po-zee-'see-on
Pulse	Pouls	Pool
Relaxation	Relâchement	Reh-'lash-mon
Rest	Repos	Reh-'po
Respiratory therapist	Spécialiste de thérapie respiratoire	Spay-'syal-eest duh té-ra-pee reh-'speer-ah-twahr'
Ribs	Côtes	Coat
Right	Droit	Drah
Sit	S'asseoir	Sahs-'swahr
Sleep	Sommeil	So-'may-uh
Slow	Lent	Lawn
Smoking	Fumer	Foo-'may
Stomach	Estomac	Eh-stome-'ah
Stop	Arrêter	Ah-reh-'tay
Take	Prendre	Prawn-'druh

Table A-23 French Words (continued)

English	French	Approximate Phonetic Pronunciation
Tent	Tente	Tawn-'tuh
Tube	Tube	Tueb
Turn	Tourner	Toor-'nay
Understand	Comprendre	Com-prawn'-druh
Up	En haut	On-oh'
Yes	Oui	Wee

Table A-24 Spanish Words

English	Spanish	Phonetic Pronunciation
Baby	Bebe	Bay-bay
Bed	Cama	Cah-ma
Blood	Sangre	San-gray
Breath	Aliento	Al-ee-'en-toe
Cannula	Canula	Khan-u-la
Chest	Pecho	'Pay-cho
Cold	Resfrio	Res-'free-o
Cough (n)	Tos	Tos
Deep	Hondo	'Awn-doe
Disease	Enfermedad	'Enn-fur-may-'dodd
Doctor	Doctor	Dock-'tore
Down	Bajo	'Ba-ho
Family	Familia	Fam-'ee-lee-ah
Fast	Rapido	'RRah-pea-doe
Head	Cabeza	Ca-'bess-a
Heart	Corazón	Cora-'sone
Hood	Caja	'Ca-ha
In	Adentro	All-'then-tro
Intensive Care Unit	Unidad de Tratamiento Intensivo	Uni-'thad day Tra-ta-'mien-toe In-ten-'see-voe
Lay	Acostarse	All-coe-'star-say

(continued)

Table A-24 Spanish Words (continued)

English	Spanish	Phonetic Pronunciation
Left	Izquierda	Is-key-'air-da
Listen to	Escuchar	Es-coo-'char
Lungs	Pulmon	Pool-'mun
Mask	Mascara	'Mas-ca-rah
Mechanical ventilation	Respiración mecánica	Re-spear-ah-see-'own mhe-'khan-ee-ca
Medication	Medicina	Med-ee-'seen-a
Mist	Vapor	Vah-'poor
Mouth	Boca	'Bo-ka
Mucous	Moco	'Moe-koe
Name	Nombre	'Nome-bray
Needle	Aguja	Ah-'goo-ha
No	No	No
No smoking	Prohibido fumar	Pro-'ee-bay fu-'mar
Normal	Normal	Nor-'mal
Nose	Nariz	Nar-'eese
Nurse (female)	Enfermera	Enn-fur-'may-rah
Out	Fuera	Ah-'fway-ra
Oxygen	Oxigeno	Awk-'see-hay-no
Oxygen tent	Tienda para oxigenación	Tea-'en-da pa-ra awk-'see-hay-no
Pain	Dolor	Doe-'lore
Patient	Paciente	Pa-see-'en-tay
Position	Posición	Po-'see-see-own
Pulse	Pulso	'Pool-so
Relaxation	Descanso	Des-'khan-so
Rest	Reposo	Re-'po-so
Respiratory therapist	Terapista de respiración	Tay-rah-'pee-sta day res-peer-a-see-'own
Ribs	Costillas	Kos-'tee-yas
Right	Derecho	Day-'ray-cho

Table A-24 Spanish Words (continued)

English	Spanish	Phonetic Pronunciation
Roll over	Darse la vuelta	'Dar-say la boo-'ell-ta
Sit	Sentarse	Sen-'tar-say
Sleep	Dormir	Door-'mear
Slow	Despacio	Des-'pa-see-o
Smoking	Fumar	Fu-'mar
Stomach	Estómago	Ex-'toe-ma-go
Stop	Alto	'Ahl-toe
Take	Tomar	Toe-'mar
Tent	Tienda	Tea-'en-da
Tube	Tubo	'Too-bow
Turn	Vuelta	Boo-'ell-ta
Understand	Entender	En-ten-'dair
Up	Arriba	Are-'ree-ba
Yes	Si	See

Table A-25 Italian Words

English	Italian	Approximate Phonetic Pronunciation
Baby	Bambino	Bahm-bee'-noe
Bed	Letto	Leh'-toe
Blood	Sangue	Sahn'-gway
Breath	Fiato	Fee-ah'-toe
Cannula	Cannula	Cahn'-noo-la
Chest	Torace	Toh-rah'-chay
Cough	Tosse	Toss'-say
Deep	Profondo	Proh-fon'-doh
Disease	Affezione	A-fetts-see-Oh'-nay
Doctor	Dottore	Doh-tor'-ray
Down	Giu	Jew
Family	Famiglia	Fah-mee'-lee-yah
Fast	Fermo	Fair'-mo

(continued)

Table A-25 Italian Words (continued)

English	Italian	Approximate Phonetic Pronunciation
Head	Testa	Test'-ah
Heart	Cuore	Kwoh'-ray
Hood	Cappuccio	Cap-poo'-chee-o
In	Entro	Ehn'-troe
Intensive Care Unit	Unita di trattamento intensivo	Oo-nit-tah di trah-tah-mehn'-toe Een-ten'-see-voh
Lay	Posare	Poe-sah'-ray
Left	Sinistro	Sih-nee-'stroe
Listen to	Ascoltare	Ah-skohl-tah'-ray
Lungs	Polmone	Pole-moan'-ay
Mask	Maschera	Mah-skeh'-rah
Mechanical ventilation	Respirazione assistita	Reh-speer-ah-tsee-'owe-nay ah-'see-stee-tah
Medicine	Medicina	Meh-dih-chee'-nah
Mist	Nebbia	Neh'-bee-yah
Mouth	Bocca	Bock'-kah
Mucous	Muco	Moo'-koh
Name	Nome	No'-may
Needle	Ago	Ah'-goe
No	No	No
No smoking	Vietato fumare	Vee-eh-tah'-toe foo-mah'-ray
Normal	Normale	Nor-mah'-lay
Nose	Naso	Nah'-soe
Nurse (female)	Infermiera	Een-fair-mee-ay'-rah
Out	Fuon	Foo-oh'-ree
Oxygen	Ossigeno	Oh-see-'jeh-noe

Table A-25 Italian Words (continued)

English	Italian	Approximate Phonetic Pronunciation
Oxygen tent	Tenda per ossigeno	'Tehn-dah pair oh-see-'jaynoh
Pain	Dolore	Doe-loe'-ray
Patient	Paziente	Pah-tsee-en'-tay
Pill	Pillola	Peel'loh-lah
Position	Posizione	Poh-zee-tsee-oh-'nay
Pulse	Polso	Pole'-soe
Relaxation	Rilassamento	Ree-lah'-sah-men'-toh
Rest	Riposo	Ree-poe'-so
Ribs	Coste	Coe'-stay
Right	Destra	Deh'-strah
Roll over	Rivoltate	Ree-vol-tah'-tay
Sit	Sedere	Say-day-'ray
Sleep	Sonno	Sonn'-noh
Slow	Lento	Lehn'-toe
Smoking	Fumare	Foo-mah'-ray
Stomach	Stomaco	Stoe-'mah-coe
Stop	Arrestare	Ahr-ress-tah'-ray
Take	Prendere	Prehn-deh'-ray
Tent	Tenda	Tehn'-dah
Tube	Tubo	Tube'-oh
Turn	Voltare	Voll-tab'-ray
Understand	Intendere	Een-ten-'day-ray
Up	Su	Soo
Yes	Si	See

Table A-26 Polish Words

English	Polish	Phonetic Pronunciation
Baby	Babe	Baa-be
Bed	Lozko	Woosh-ko
Blood	Krew	Krrev
Breath	Dech	Deh
Breathe	Oddychac	Awd-deh-hach
Chest	Skrzunic	K-shoo-neats
Cough	Kaszel	Ka-shell
Deep	Gleboki	Gwem-bo-key
Doctor	Dohor	Dok-tore
Down	Dolle	Dough-leh
Family	Rodzine	Ro-gee-na
Fast	Szybki	Ship-kee
Head	Glowa	Gwo-va
Heart	Serce	Selt-ze
Hood	Kaptur	Kop-tour
In	Wewnatrz	Vev-noonch
Lay down	Skladac	Squaq-datch
Lay on	Nakladac	Naw-qua-dach
Left	Lewy	Levy
Listen to	Kogos	Ko-gush
Lungs	Pluco	Pwu-tzo
Mask	Maska	Maw-ska
Medicine	Medycyna	Med-et-sin-a
Mist	Mgla	Meh-gwa
Mouth	Usta	Uh-stah
Needle	Igla	EE-gwan
No	Nie	Nyeh
No smoking	Nie wolno palic	Nyeh vol-no pa-leech
Normal	Normalny	Nan-mawl-ne

(continued)

Table A-26 Polish Words (continued)

English	Polish	Phonetic Pronunciation
Nose	Nos	Noss
Nurse	Nianka	Knee-yan-ka
Out	Na zew natrz	Na Zev Nunch
Oxygen	Tlen	Tel-en
Pain	Bol	Bole
Patient	Cierpliwy	Cher-plea-vy
Position	Posada	Paw-sa-da
Pulse	Puls	Pulls
Relaxation	Oslabienie	Os-wa-bee-yen-ye
Respiratory therapist	Oddechowy terapia	Awd-deh-ho-vy terr-aw-pea-a
Rib	Zebra	Zeh-bra
Right	Prawy	Prah-vy
Roll over	Odwrocic	Owd-lvu-cheech
Sit	Siedziec	Sheh-jetch
Sleep	Spac	Spahch
Slow	Powolny	Po-vol-ne
Smoker	Palacz	Pa-lech
Stomach	Zoladek	Zaw-won-deck
Stop	Zatkac	Katch
Take	Brac	Bratch
Tent	Namlot	Nem-watt
Tube	Rura	Ru-rah
Turn	Vi obracac	Vee O-brah-chatch
Understand	Rozumiec	Roh-zoom-meech
Up	Gorze	Goo-zech
Yes	Tak	Tuk

Table A-26 German Words

English	German	Phonetic Pronunciation
Baby	Baby	Baa-be
Bed	Bett	Bet
Blood	Blut	Blool
Breath	Atem	Ah'-tem
Breathe	Atmen	Aht'-men
Cannula	Kanüle	Kahn'-oohluh
Chest	Brust	Broost
Cough	Husten	Hoo'-stun
Deep	Tief	Teef
Disease	übel	Ooh'-buhl
Doctor	Doktor	Dock'-tohr
Down	Nieder	nee'-der
Family	Familie	Fah'-meelyah
Fast	Fest	Fest
Head	Kopf	Cawpf
Heart	Herz	Hairts
In	In	In
Intensive Care Unit	Intensivstation	In-ten-'siv-'stahts-'ee-ohn
Lay	Legen	Lay-'gehn
Left	Links	Lihnks
Listen to	Hören	'Hœren
Lungs	Lunge	Luhn'-guh
Mask	Maske	'Mah-skuh
Mechanical ventilation	Assistielte atmung	As-sis-steer'-the aht'-moong
Medication	Arznei	Arts'-nye
Mouth	Mund	Moont
Mucous	Schleim	Shlime
Name	Name	Nahm'-uh
Needle	Nadel	Nah'-dul

Table A-26 German Words (continued)

English	German	Phonetic Pronunciation
No	Nein	Nine
No smoking	Rauchen verboten	rou-'khen fair-boh-'ten
Normal	Normal	Norm-al'
Nose	Nase	Nah-'suh
Nurse	Kraukenschwester	Krahn-ken-schwehst-'er
Out	Aus	Ows
Oxygen	Sauerstoff	Zou-'er -shtoff
Oxygen tent	Sauerstoffzelt	Zou-'er-shtoff-'tsehlt
Pain	Schmerz	Shmairts
Patient	Patient	Patsi-'ent
Position	Stellung	Shtehl'-oong
Pulse	Puls	Pools
Relaxation	Entspannung	Ehnt-spah'-noong
Rest	Pause	Pou'-suh
Ribs	Rippen	Rih'-pehn
Right	Recht	Rehkt
Sit	Sitzen	Zit-'sen
Sleep	Schlaf	Shlahf
Slow	Nachgehen	Nahkh-'gay-ehn
Smoking	Rauchen	Rou'-khen
Stomach	Magen	Mah'-gehn
Stop	Halten	Hahl-'ten
Take	Nehmen	Nay-'men
Tent	Zelt	Tselt
Tube	Rohr	Roar
Turn	Wenden	Ven-'den
Understand	Verstehen	Fair-stay-'en
Up	Auf	Ouf
Yes	Ja	Yah

■ POSTURAL DRAINAGE POSITIONS

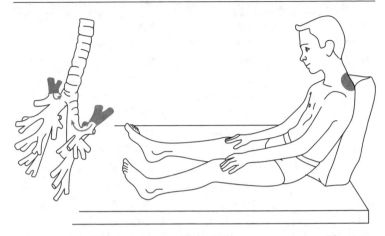

Figure A-1 Upper lobes, apical segment. Patient sits and leans back on a pillow at a 30-degree angle against the therapist. Clap between the clavicle and the top of the scapula on each side.

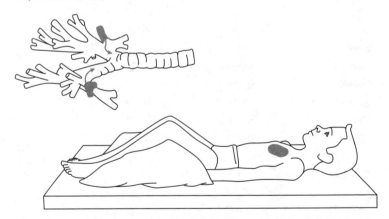

Figure A-2 Upper lobes, anterior segment. Patient lies on his back with knees flexed. Clap between the clavicle and nipple on each side.

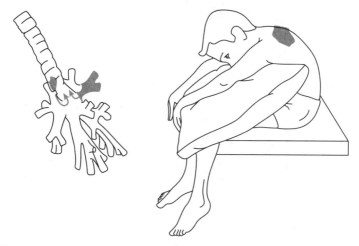

Figure A-3 Upper lobes, posterior segment. Patient leans forward over a folded pillow at a 30-degree angle. Clap over the upper back on both sides.

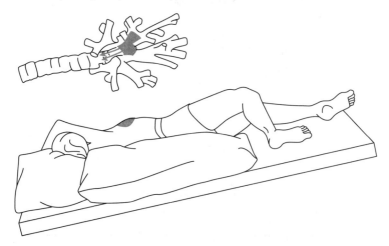

Figure A-4 Right middle lobe, lateral segment; medial segment. Bed is elevated 14 in. (about 15 degrees). The patient lies head down on the left side and rotates one quarter turn backward. The knees should be flexed. Clap over the right nipple. In females with breast development or tenderness, use cupped hand with heel of hand under armpit and fingers extending forward beneath the breast.

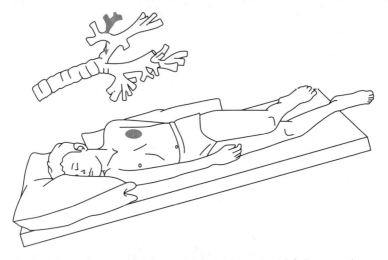

Figure A-5 Lingular segment, left upper lobe, superior segment, inferior segment. Patient in a head-down position on the right side and rotated one quarter turn backward. Clap over the left nipple.

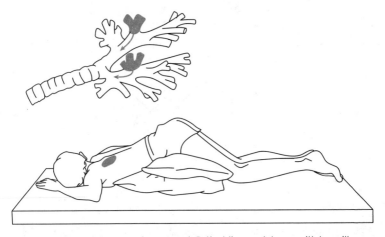

Figure A-6 Lower lobes, superior segment. Patient lies on abdomen with two pillows under the hips. Clap over the middle part of the back at the tip of the scapula on either side of the spine.

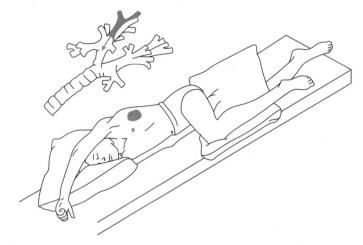

Figure A-7 Lower lobes, anterior basal segments. The foot of the bed is elevated 18 in. (about 30 degrees). The patient lies on his side with a pillow between the knees. Clap over the lower ribs just beneath the axilla.

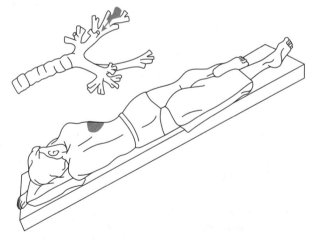

Figure A-8 Lower lobes, lateral basal segments. The foot of the bed is elevated 18 in. (approximately 30 degrees). The patient lies on his abdomen, head down, and rotates one quarter turn upward from a prone position. The upper leg is flexed over a pillow for support. Clap over the uppermost portion of the lower ribs.

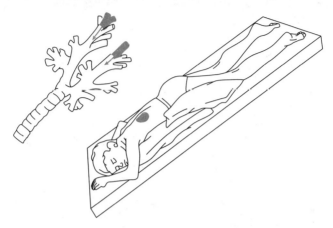

Figure A-9 Lower lobes. posterior basal segments. The foot of the bed is elevated 18 in. (about 30 degrees). The patient lies on his abdomen, head down, with a pillow under the hips. Clap over the lower ribs close to the spine on each side.

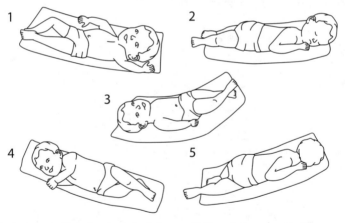

Figure A-10 Positions for chest physiotherapy. (1) The anterior segment of the upper lobes is drained in a supine position at a 30-degree upright angle. (2) Drain the apical segment of the right lung while the infant lies on his left side at a 30-degree upright angle. (3) The posterior segment of the right upper lobe is drained in a prone position with the right side elevated 45 degrees. (4) Drain the anterior segment of the upper lobe in a supine position.

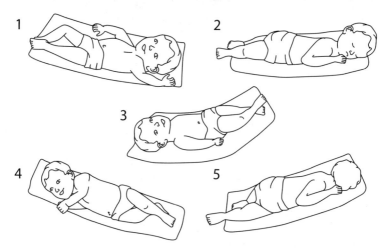

Figure A-11 (1) The right middle lobe is drained at a 15-degree, head-down angle, with a 45-degree rotation to the left. To drain the lingula, rotate to the right. (2) The superior segments of the lower lobes drain in a prone position. (3) Drain the anterior basal segments of the lower lobes at a 30-degree, head-down position. (4) The basal segments of the lower lobe are drained at a 30-degree, head-down position while the infant is lying on his side. (5) The posterior basal segments of the lower lobes are drained at a 30-degree, head-down prone position.

INDEX

Note: Italicized page locators indicate a figure; tables are noted with a *t*.